The New

5:2 Diet

Cookbook

2017 Edition
Now 800 Calories a Day

Jacqueline Whitehart

PEPIK BOOKS

Pepik Books

York

www.52recipes.co.uk

A catalogue record for this book is
available from the British Library.

ISBN: 978-1-5448374-1-3

The New 5:2 Diet

The Recipes

New Introduction for 2017

Welcome to The New 5:2 Diet

Choose between the traditional 500 calories a day and the new rules: 800 calories a day but with an enforced 14 hour overnight fast.

Since the principles of 5:2 Dieting were popularized in 2012, our knowledge and understanding of how the fasting phenomenon affects our weight-loss and our bodies has matured.

If you're someone for whom The 5:2 Diet held an appeal the first time round, but found you couldn't sustain it due to the very restricted calories then this new book might just be for you.

Find the right way to follow The 5:2 Diet for you by taking the fantastic new quiz.

Explore what you can and can't eat to successfully lose weight.

Learn more about how an overnight fast can benefit your health.

Discover over 100 new and revised recipes, designed to be simple, filling and tasty.

I'm excited to be getting back into The 5:2 in 2017. The new calorie allowance of 800 calories is tempting me back again. I gave up on the diet a few years ago because I couldn't cope with just 500 calories, I was dreading my diet days and I was struggling to lose weight.

The New 5:2 Diet is for you, for me, for everyone. It's easier to stick to than ever before. Why? Its rules are so simple, it's not too restrictive AND because you only diet two days a week. For five full days you are not on a diet. Because you know that following each day on which you diet you can eat normally the motivation to complete the diet day without giving in to temptation is high. When you see yourself losing weight and still continuing to eat as normal 5 days a week it's easy to find the strength to carry on.

With the new rules, you'll find that The New 5:2 Diet is even easier to follow.

Join me and let's lose weight together.

Jacqueline

X

Weekly new recipes on **www.52recipes.co.uk**

Facebook **@52DietRecipes**

Twitter **@52DietRecipes**

The 5:2 Diet and Me

Back in 2012 I produced the first ever 5:2 Diet Recipe Book and it changed my life. A book of recipes, written from the heart by a very normal Mum, became a Top 5 Amazon best-seller and led to a book deal with a major publisher and a series of new books about diet and healthy eating.

I came across the diet quite by chance and was so impressed by the claimed health benefits that I decided it was worth a try. Straight away I saw the benefits. Immediate weight-loss and increased energy. I was producing recipes for myself and carefully calorie-counting them. I started to share the recipes and then it all went a little bit crazy! Everyone wanted to do the 5:2 Diet but couldn't work out how to eat so few calories and not starve. And that's where the idea for the Recipe Book was born.

For the next two years I lived and breathed the 5:2 Diet: producing new books, running a popular blog and becoming an expert in the field. But as with all new things, my interest waned when I found I could no longer follow the diet. I found the diet days increasingly challenging and I stopped losing weight…in fact I started to gain weight. That's when I fell out of love with the 5:2 Diet. And although I still shared calorie-counted recipes via my blog www.52recipes.co.uk, I stopped following the diet entirely.

Fast forward to 2017.

Still writing. Still cooking. Still dieting. And I heard something new and exciting. The 5:2 Diet was changing. 500 calories was being upped to 800 calories…but with a catch. Your diet day has to include a 14 hour complete fast.

The science behind this is so interesting and stems from the fact that now thousands of people have followed the diet, we can see what works and what doesn't...for the majority of people.

But everyone is so different. How can we make a diet plan that fits us all? Quite simply we can't. And that is what this new book on the 5:2 Diet will explore. There is no 'right' way to follow the 5:2 Diet: you need to find the way that suits you.

I have been inspired to start the 5:2 Diet again and I'd love you to try it with me. I hope this book will show you the best path to follow the diet. Try the quiz. Find your plan. And use the healthy, tasty and filling recipes to make your diet days easy.

The New Golden Rules

Let's cut to the chase: there are three steps that we will be following in The New 5:2 Diet Plan. Follow these rules and you will lose weight, feel healthier and look great.

- *Two Days of 800 Calories – eat only 800 calories over 2 meals – on two non-consecutive days per week.*
- *On your 800 calorie days, include a 14 hour fast either the night before or the night after your diet day.*
- *Eat normally but healthily on the other five days.*

Looks simple doesn't it? That's because it is! It's really simple and easy to follow, so read on and I will guide you through each of the three rules.

1 Two days of 800 Calories

Two days a week you follow a calorie-restricted diet, that's 800 calories for men and women eaten over two meals.

- Breakfast or Lunch 300 Calories
- Dinner 500 Calories

The days are non-consecutive.

2 Fast for 14 hours at the start or the end of your 800 Calorie Day

That means either:

Starting the night before and counting 14 hours from the last food you ate the day before

Eg: Finish dinner at 7pm on Sunday, eat breakfast at 9am on Monday

OR

Finish the diet day with a 14 hour fast. Count 14 hours from the end of an early dinner on your diet day and fast until the next morning.

Eg. Finish dinner at 5.30pm on Monday, eat breakfast at 7.30am on Tuesday

3 Eat normally but healthily on the other five days

If you have followed The 5:2 Diet before you will be familiar with the term 'feast' day, but that's something that trips people up time and time again. This is because most of us, if told we can eat what we like, go a bit mad.

The five non-fast days are normal and healthy days. However, they are not diet days and we do not count calories.

- Enjoy your food and don't count the calories.
- Eat three healthy meals a day.
- Do NOT snack between meals and avoid processed food.

Cut out the rubbish. Keep the following items to a very bare minimum:

- biscuits (cookies) and cakes
- Crisps (potato chips)
- Non-diet fizzy drinks
- Chocolate bars and sweets (candies)
- Beer, lager and cider

If you follow these steps, you will have plenty of scope for tasty plates of food without excluding any food group, and it means that you will be able to have delicious pasta, bread, desserts and, of course, a glass or two of wine.

Remember that the recipes in this book are not just for diet days; they are perfect for your normal days too. Just add some extra carbohydrates, such as rice or potatoes, if necessary and make sure you eat three balanced meals every day.

What if I like the old rules?

If you like the old rules – 500 calories for women, 600 calories for men – then of course you should stick to them. These new rules are intended for lapsed 5:2ers (of which there are many thousands) and for those who found they couldn't survive on just 500 calories per day. By tweaking the diet and allowing 60% more calories, the 5:2 Plan is more sustainable long-term.

How can you eat more calories and still lose (almost) as much weight?

This seems to be a critical question for many 5:2ers, both old and new. The revised 5:2 increases the allowed calories on a diet day from 500 to 800. That's a 60% increase for women. How can the diet work as well?

There are three aspects to this that I will look at individually:

14 Hour Fast

Firstly, the addition of an enforced 14 hour fast. This is a key part of the new diet and goes hand in hand with the increased calorie allowance.

One of the problems with the original 5:2 Plan was that it wasn't really a fast at all. You have your meals at the same time as normal. It is just a very calorie restricted diet – not a fast. Some of the major health benefits of the 5:2 Diet come from the fasting element: where you do not consume any calories for an extended period of time. A lot of the original research into the health benefits of the 5:2 Diet come from fasting, not calorie restriction. Enforcing a strict fast into the diet triggers a hormonal and fat-loss reaction in the body. When you diet through calorie-restriction, the body will always use the simplest energy stores first. This means that you will always burn off the food you have just eaten rather than the fat on your hips. When you enforce the fast, you enter a semi-fasting state and your blood glucose levels fall. This triggers the release of metabolic fuels from the body's store of fat. Put simply, we can eat more calories as long as we are stricter with the 14 hour fast.

Over-eating on non-diet Days

Another problem with the original 5:2 Diet was that the day after a diet day was a 'eat all you want' day. And a lot of people got a lot of cravings on their normal days that they satisfied by eating very badly. While not setting rules for the non-restricted days of the diet, the increased calories consumed on the diet days should counteract the 'need to feed' on the normal days. Also, the act of fasting (as opposed to consuming low calorie) also puts a break on increased consumption that should last several days.

To be successful at weight-loss on the 5:2 Diet, we should not obsess about food on normal days but we should try and stick to the following:

- reduce processed food and empty calories

- don't snack between meals
- make it, don't buy it

Finding the 5:2 Diet too hard

Many people, myself included, gave up on The 5:2. This isn't because it doesn't work – it does! But it's simply because sticking to 500 calories is just too difficult – especially in the long-term. If you dread your diet days or find excuse after excuse to skip the diet days then you're going to give up. It's going to be another failure to add to your list. My problem was both of these combined plus a sense of every little thing getting on top of me on a diet day. So it wasn't so much that I was 'hangry' (hungry angry), more that I couldn't cope with the normal everyday little things. That's not a way to live (even just two days a week) so I stopped. But I'm looking at this now – as I suspect many of you are too – and thinking 'Yes I could do this'.

So let's stop talking about it and make a plan, cook some delicious low-calorie food, and start losing weight.

The Different 5:2 Plans

Plan A: ORIGINAL

This is the original 500 calorie (600 for men) plan. You eat 3 meals a day with no extended fast BUT you have to keep to the lower calorie limit.

We're working on the theory that 'If it ain't broke don't fix it.'

Perhaps you've done 5:2 before and are not one of those people who gets irritable on the lower calorie regime. Or maybe you just have to eat breakfast and can't imagine going for a significant time without food.

Obviously how you divide the calories between your meals is up to you. But I would suggest:

100 for breakfast, 100-200 for lunch and 200-300 for dinner

Your **breakfast** could be a small banana, natural yogurt perhaps or an egg.

Lunch is also light and is likely to be either a soup or a salad.

Dinner is relatively normal and should contain some good quality protein: chicken, fish or beans. You will however have to cut back on the carbs to keep within the calorie restrictions. You'll find plenty of the recipes in this book will be less than 300 calories, especially if you take out the potatoes, rice or similar carbs.

Plan B: NEW

This is the 800 calorie plan with a 14 hour fast from the night before. You will eat 2 meals: Late Breakfast/Brunch or Lunch followed by a proper dinner.

With this plan, you get the hard bit out of the way in the morning, have a satisfying lunch and then a completely normal dinner – carbs and all!

Again the calorie split is up to you, but you shouldn't eat more than twice in the day. My recommended calorie split is 300 for breakfast/lunch and 500 for dinner. You might also want to split dinner into the main course and a small sweet treat (eg. Yogurt, fruit or chocolate).

The 14 hour fast works like this:

You don't consume any calories for a 14 hour period overnight. This means no calories at all for 14 hours. Calorie free drinks (both hot and cold) are allowed and encouraged during this time.

Depending on what works best for you and your situation you can do the following (or anything in between)

Start early the night before. Eat your dinner early. Make a note of what time you finish – this could be 6pm for example. Also, make sure you don't have any snacks or calorific drinks (including alcohol) after this time. When you wake up in the morning don't eat first thing. You can have coffee or tea but without milk or sugar. I like a green tea as this is caffeinated but has no calories. You can have your substantial breakfast (including coffee or tea with milk) as soon as the 14 hours have elapsed. So if you finished your dinner the night before at 6pm, then you can have breakfast as early as 8am.

If you don't want to think about your diet day the night before your diet – that's fair enough. But remember you will have to wait quite a while before you have anything to eat the next morning. If you're someone who can easily skip breakfast then this would work really well for you. If you have your last nibble of food / sip of wine at 9pm, then you must save your self for a late breakfast / early lunch at 11am the next day. Same rules apply re tea and coffee. Tea and coffee and caffeinated drinks are all allowed before you eat but can't contain any calories.

Plan C: ALTERNATIVE

Plan C is an alternative 800 calorie plan where you do the 14 hour fast at the END of your diet day. This will work well for you if you want to keep your diet within one day. And also if you prefer to have 3 meals a day yet still be allowed 800 calories.

For this plan to work you eat either Breakfast and Lunch (totalling 300 calories) or just Lunch (totalling 300 calories) followed by an EARLY 500 calorie Dinner.

The key to making the Alternative Plan work is the early dinner on your diet day. The following day, just make sure you don't eat until 14 hours has passed. So if you have your early dinner on your diet day and finish by 5.30pm, you'll be able to eat breakfast as normal the next day at 7.30am.

Suggested Alternative Plan
Breakfast – 100 calories eg. A small banana, natural yogurt, half a grapefruit, an egg

Lunch – 200 calories (or skip breakfast and have 300 cals)
Early dinner – 500 calories

Find the right 5:2 Diet Plan for you and your lifestyle

If you're struggling to work out which of these 5:2 Plans works for you, then take the quick quiz to discover which one fits you best.

What 5:2 Diet Plan would suit me best?

1 Have you followed The 5:2 Diet before?

A Yes and still follow it successfully now

B Yes but lapsed

C No I've never tried it

2 Would you say you had a sweet tooth?

A I enjoy sweet things but can live without them

B Yes, absolutely I love sweet things and eat them several times a day

C No

3 How often do you eat bread, pasta, cakes or biscuits?

A 3 times or more a day

B Once or twice a day

C Less than once a day

4 How many times do you eat a day?

A 3 meals a day

B Sometimes skip meals

C Snack between meals at least once a day

5 Do you ever feel weak and wobbly between meals?

A Yes often

B Occasionally but only if I don't eat right, or go a long time without eating

C Never

6 How late do you eat in the evening?

A Early (before 6pm)

B Mid (6-8pm)

C Late (after 8pm)

7 How do you feel about breakfast?

A Absolutely essential

B Normally have it but could eat later or skip it

C Take it or leave it

8 When do you eat breakfast?

A Very Early (before 7am)

B Early (before 8am)

C Mid (8-9am)

D After 9am/Don't eat breakfast

Add up your scores using the following key:

1. A – score 0, B – score 3, C – score 5; 2. A – 0, B – 3, C – 5; 3. A – 5, B – 3, C – 3; 4. A – 0, B – 3, C – 3; 5. A – 5, B – 3, C – 3; 6. A – 3, B – 3, C – 5; 7. A – 0, B – 3, C – 3; 8. A – 0, B – 0, C – 3, D – 5;

Score 0-14

If you score between 0-14 then you are an ORIGINAL and should follow Plan A. That's 500 calories (600 Men) and 3 meals a day.

Score 15-29

If you score between 15-29 then you are a NEW and should follow Plan B. That's 800 calories per day over 2 meals with a 14 hour fast overnight before your diet day.

Score 30-40

If you score between 30-40 then you are an ALTERNATIVE and should follow Plan C. That's 800 calories per day over 2 or 3 meals with a 14 hour fast at the end of your diet day.

Let's Get Started

Now you know the basics it's time to get started and think about your first fast day.

Are you fit and well and ready to lose some weight?

The first thing to think about is what days would be most suitable for a fast. Remember, you need two days a week with at least one rest day in between. You can have a set routine and pick the same days every week or pick and choose. The diet is extremely flexible and is designed to fit in around you and not the other way round.

What days do you normally fast?

'Tuesdays and Thursdays. My husband is out so I don't have to worry about catering for anyone else on those days.'
Patricia

Monday is a common day to start as most people want to enjoy their food at the weekend and are ready to start the new week with good resolutions.

'I like to fast on a Monday, to get rid of that weekend bloat, and on a Thursday, in preparation for the weekend bloat!'
Jocelyn

Take a look at your schedule for the week and rule out any days where you have social engagements, especially involving food.

'My fast days are variable, depending on what I am doing that week. It changes from week to week.'

Kat

Look at this as the greatest asset of the diet. Imagine going out for dinner with friends, not worrying about what you eat and even having a dessert and wine, and all the time losing weight. Do the planning, do the fast days and then for five days a week, don't diet. Especially when you are first starting out, your diet days should be the least social days on your calendar. Ideally, they should also be busy days or work days, as you want to be distracted from food and away from the kitchen as much as possible. The only restriction on your fast days is that you must have a rest day between fasts.

Your first fast day will probably be the hardest as your body needs time to adjust to the new regime. So make sure you pick your days wisely when you start out. For the first two weeks you need to give careful consideration to when you fast as there is a possibility that you will feel lightheaded, grumpy and perhaps get a headache as well as feel properly hungry. Don't worry or be alarmed. There are plenty of tips here to deal with all these things. After the first two weeks of fast days, you will see it getting considerably easier. Focus on the fact that it's only one day.

Setting targets

Before you start you need to take your starting weight. Don't think about it too much – everyone's starting weight is high, otherwise you wouldn't be thinking about your diet. Think positively. Think how good you will feel when you start losing weight.

A few tips about weighing yourself

Don't worry about only weighing yourself once a week. You should weigh yourself when you like, just try not to do it every day as your weight can go up as well as down. We only care about the downward trend.

Ladies, be aware that your bodily cycle will have an impact on your weight. You may put on weight the week before your period and may also find fasting harder during this time. Try and stick with it and make allowances for your cycle if you find you haven't lost as much weight as you would like. I would recommend weighing yourself the morning after your second fast day of the week. If you fast on Mondays and Wednesdays, then Thursday morning before breakfast or a drink and after you have been to the toilet is when you will be at your lightest. If you can, use this as your weekly weigh-in to see if you have lost weight and hit your target.

How much weight should you aim to lose?

This will depend entirely on your starting weight and fitness. If you have got more to lose, you will lose weight faster and can set a higher target. If you are quite close to your target weight and already reasonably fit, you won't be quite as quick but you will still lose weight.

The target for your weight loss should be between 1 and 3lb per week. This is not a crash diet and you should only be aiming to lose weight in a safe and sensible way.

As a general guide, if you are just fasting but not exercising you should aim to lose 1lb per week. If you are fasting, exercising and staying healthy on your normal days then you could potentially see a weight loss of 2–3lb per week.

If you have more than two stone to lose then your target could be potentially higher than that.

Keeping yourself hydrated

On a 5:2 Diet Day you'll find that you are naturally more thirsty than normal. Drinking water will actually help fill you up and ward off any headaches.

Water and more water

I know it's boring but water is refreshing and good for you.

Sparkling water with ice and lemon

Make a glass of water so much more of an event by serving chilled sparkling mineral water with ice and lemon. This also works with still mineral water and even tap water.

Fresh lime soda

This is another way to jazz up a simple glass of water naturally. Place several ice cubes in a long tall glass. Halve a fresh lime and cut off one generous slice. Squeeze the rest of the lime juice into the glass. Add your choice of still or sparkling water and top with the slice of lime. This is extremely refreshing and only adds 2 calories so knock yourself out!

Fruit teas and more

Apart from your normal tea and coffee, you may find a fruit tea, or a chamomile, peppermint or similar is just the ticket when you want something un-caffeinated and warming. There are so many to choose from these days so stick to your favourite if you have one or try a selection if you're new to them.

Exercise

If you exercise hard on your diet days you may feel light-headed or find the hunger pangs difficult to bear. So take a break and make sure the only exercise you do is a very gentle. Gentle exercise is relaxing and makes you feel great. The simplest of all is a half an hour walk. But a gentle swim or a yoga class would be perfect too.

Why is simple walking so beneficial?

Walking is a fantastic exercise for many reasons. Perhaps the most important is that it lowers your stress hormones. This not only makes you feel better but also encourages your body to burn fat, not sugar.

Your metabolic response to walking means that each time you walk (or swim or do yoga) you are reducing your insulin resistance by a tiny bit and enhancing your ability to burn fat. So never dismiss walking as 'not proper exercise', embrace and enjoy it.

(Genuine) Frequently Asked Questions

These are all genuine questions that people have asked via Facebook **www.facebook.com/52DietRecipes** or Twitter **@52DietRecipes**. If you've got a question that's not listed here, I'd love to help if I can.

Q: Can I have caffeinated drinks?

A: Yes

Do you drink coffee or tea or colas regularly every day? You are definitely not alone. I do NOT advise you to give them up, even on your diet days. Why? Because caffeine withdrawal is likely to give you headaches and make your fasting days miserable and harder. So unless you have other reasons to give up caffeine just work out your normal consumption and make sure you count all the calories you have in your caffeinated drinks.

There are lots of ways to get your normal caffeine hit without adding any calories. Black tea and coffee - great. Diet colas/energy drinks – if you must. The calories in these drinks are insignificant.

But if your preferred drink is tea or coffee with milk then don't cut it out. Just make sure you count the calories in each cup. You could also consider shifting to skimmed milk which has 35 cals per 100ml as opposed to semi-skimmed which has 49 cals per 100ml.

Remember: you can't drink tea or coffee with milk during the 14 hour fast period. You'll either have to drink them black or simply wait until you pass the 14 hour threshold.

Q: What if I only want to eat once a day?

A: Of course. This can be incorporated into the 500 cal and 800 cal programme

If you feel you can cut back to just one meal a day then this is a great way to do the 5:2 Diet. You should have one meal - an early evening meal or a late lunch. If you are just starting out then I would recommend leaving this option for a few weeks as your body gets used to fewer calories.

The great thing about the one meal a day option is that the 14 hour fast is already built into the plan. Plus the main meal is a really satisfying and filling meal. Your main course will include carbohydrates, protein and fat and will probably be around 400 to 500 calories. Then if you wish, you can add some fruit, yogurt or chocolate to give yourself a treat afterwards. Don't feel you have to use all your calories exactly. Anything between 500 to 800 is fine. Just don't go overboard and start on the biscuits.

Q: Should I exercise as normal?

A: Not on your diet days

Sometimes you will find that you have to do exercise on your diet day. The problem with exercising is that it burns calories and makes you hungry, meaning that you are more likely to struggle with your diet day. Sadly you cannot add on the calories that you burn during exercise to your calorie intake for the day. If you do need to exercise on a diet day, try to do it before you eat in the morning and make sure it's low intensity. Light exercise in the evening can also be a distraction from hunger. Try to avoid exercising in the afternoon as this will make you very hungry and most likely to falter.

Q: What is the best type of exercise to do on my normal days?

A: Any sweaty exercise that gets your heart rate up

I would recommend any aerobic exercise that increases your breathing and heart rate as being best for weight loss. Walking, jogging, cycling, swimming or tennis are all good to get your heart rate up. Try to exercise three times a week for at least 45 minutes each time.

Q: What about alcoholic drinks?

A: Not on your diet days

Alcoholic drinks contain plenty of calories and will probably make you feel light-headed on your diet days so it's worth steering clear of alcoholic drinks on these days. An alcoholic drink will also affect will-power and your ability to avoid extra calories. Of course you're free to do what you want on the other 5 days.

Q: What should I eat on normal (non-diet) days?

A: Healthy normal food with a few treats

If you avoid junk food, you can almost what you like and really enjoy it. This is your reward for the fast day before. Your body will regulate itself and even on the day after a fast day you'll at most eat 10% - 15% more than normal.

Be aware that on the first day after a fast day the breakfast that you've been looking forward to may be a bit of a let down. You'll be surprised that you cannot manage to eat as much as you thought you wanted. You may also feel rather tired and lethargic that first feast day. This is just your body compensating for the fast day. As your body gets used to fasting this won't happen and feast days will be trouble-free.

Q: What if your plans change and you suddenly find yourself 'out' on a diet day

A: Don't panic!

You have got two choices. Do you break the diet or not? Having a drink and breaking the diet would mean that the effort you have put in during the day would be lost and you'd have to schedule another diet day later in the week. If it's the evening and you have already got through most of the day, is it really worth giving up on the diet day? You could have a water, a diet coke or diet tonic water without adding any extra calories.

Q: What if you're starving and there's nothing in the cupboards

A: Eggs, baked beans and soups are your friends here.

All are filling and you should find the calorie content on the box. If you don't have any of these in your house, all will be available from your nearest supermarket or convenience store.

Q: If you find a diet day is proving next to impossible

A: Sometimes this happens to the best of us.

For all sorts of reasons – stress, hormonal, lack of sleep – we can find a diet day particularly hard. You are allowed to give up on a day if it is truly dreadful.

It is always worth assessing what is causing it to be so hard and trying to see if it is worth pushing on through. Late afternoon is often a time when we feel at our weakest. If you can bring your evening meal forward or have a small snack at that time, you may find you get over the hump. Remember that the sacrifices you have made already during the day will be wasted if you stop.

Try counting the number of hours until bedtime and make sure you get an early night.

If you give up entirely on a diet day, don't beat yourself up about it. Allow yourself tomorrow off and re-attempt the following day. If you still manage to fit two diet days into your week, then the week has been a success.

Q: What if you are going on holiday
A: Take a well-earned rest.

If you have been dieting for weeks beforehand, then I would say that it is time to relax and enjoy your hard work. To avoid putting on too much weight, try to still be sensible when you can. Eat a big breakfast (especially if it's free!), eat healthy snacks or a light lunch and enjoy your dinner.

Q: What if you're cooking for other (unsympathetic!) people
A: Cook the same meal for everyone

If you have got a partner or family who are not dieting then you need to make sure you can accommodate everyone's needs without much fuss. The easiest way to deal with this common problem is to cook the same meal for everyone. Just serve everyone else's meal with plenty of extra carbohydrates. If it's not possible to all eat the same thing, then at the very least try to eat at the same time. There's nothing worse than watching other people eat when you're starving.

Q: What if you feel that your weight loss has plateaued

A: It is natural for your weight loss to level out after a few weeks on The 5:2 Diet.

The high weight loss that you experience when you start the diet can only be maintained for two to three weeks.

After that, at the same time as it gets easier and you get into a rhythm, the weight loss will diminish. This is normal and healthy. The extreme early weight loss cannot be maintained. If you have a lot of weight to lose, then you will hopefully find that the weight loss flattens out at about 0.9kg (2lb) a week. If you are nearer your target weight, your expected weight loss will be about 0.5kg (1lb) a week.

If you are not losing any weight while still following the diet plan, then you should look at what you are eating on the five normal days. You may be eating too much. Indeed this is the most likely cause of a plateau. Make a food diary for your healthy days and be a bit stricter with yourself. Most importantly steer away from the biscuit tin and any junk food.

How to add treats to the menu without busting the plan

If you're like me and love a little something sweet after your meal then you should consider cutting back your main meal calories by about 100 and allow yourself something sweet to finish off.

The sweet treat doesn't need to be unhealthy – we are talking fruit, natural yogurt or a little bit of chocolate. Adding some natural sugar in in this way can help you feel satiated and 'finished'.

Here's a list of some healthy sweet treats and their calories. Simply have a few less calories as part of your main course to fit it in.

Note: These 'healthy snacks' should be consumed as part of lunch or dinner not on their own.

Fruit

Small banana - 76 cals

Orange - 52 cals

Satsuma - 18 cals

Bunch of red grapes (10-15) - 60 cals

10 strawberries (100g) - 27 cals

Apple - 47 cals

Kiwi – 42 cals

Half a Grapefruit - 42 cals

Yogurt, Jelly and Custard

100g Natural yogurt – 82 cals

100g Natural yogurt with a wisp (1/2 tsp) of honey – 105 cals

125g pot custard – 124 cals

115g sugar-free jelly pot – 5 cals

Chocolate

6 squares (20g) dark chocolate -120 cals

Plate Fillers

If you have calculated your calories for a meal and have found you have a few to spare then this is the place to look. Generally if you have got 100 or more calories to play with then you could add some good carbohydrates, like rice or new potatoes. If you have got 50–100 calories to spare, consider adding a salad or mixed vegetables. And don't despair if you have got less than 50 calories left over, you can still have a plate full of carefully chosen green veg or salad leaves.

New potatoes go well with chicken or any dish with a sauce – 200g (7oz) new potatoes have 140 calories. That's about 4 small potatoes in their skins. Pop them on the scales to make sure you have the right amount.

Brown rice has a dense nutty flavour and is incredibly filling. A 40g (scant ¼ cup) portion (that's dry weight) has 143 calories. Note that brown rice takes about 30 minutes to cook – check the packet instructions. An easy alternative is precooked microwaveable brown rice. Try Tilda steamed microwave rice – half a 250g (9oz) packet has 158 calories.

Basmati rice is also a good carbohydrate and cooks in 10 minutes. I use a microwave rice cooker and it's a breeze. Again it is worth weighing the rice to make sure you get the correct amount. A 40g (scant ¼ cup) serving (dry weight) has 144 calories.

Couscous is a great low-calorie grain. It's extremely easy to cook – just pour over boiling water, cover and leave to cook for about 10 minutes. A 40g (scant ¼ cup) (dry weight) portion has 91 calories.

Quinoa differs from other grains in that it mixes carbohydrate and protein. It is therefore particularly good with a vegetarian dish. You cook it similarly to rice and it takes about 15 minutes. A 40g (scant ¼ cup) dry weight serving has 124 calories.

Bulgur wheat makes an unusual addition to your plate. Cook according to the packet instructions (normally about 20 minutes). A 40g (scant ¼ cup) dry weight portion has 141 calories.

A small (150g/5oz) baked **sweet potato** has 130 calories. I find it easiest to microwave the sweet potato first for 3–4 minutes and then bake in a preheated oven at 200C/180C fan/400F for about 10 minutes. Don't forget to prick your sweet potato several times before cooking.

A slice of **wholemeal (wholewheat) bread** is perhaps the quickest addition to your plate. A medium slice from a sliced loaf has about 65 calories. Check the packet for the calorific content of your bread as it can vary considerably.

Salads and Mixed Vegetables

If you have got less than 100 calories to spare then consider a salad or mixed veg on the side. Please note that average calorie counts have been given for generic foods (tomatoes, apples, eggs, etc.), but these will vary according to their individual size and weight.

Salad 58 calories

1 Little Gem (Boston) lettuce, shredded (20 cals)

1 × 5cm (2in) piece cucumber, thinly sliced (10 cals)

2 medium tomatoes, sliced (28 cals)

Mixed veg 80 calories

1 carrot, peeled and sliced (35 cals)

50g (1¾oz) fine green beans (12 cals)

50g (1¾oz) frozen peas (frozen weight) (33 cals)

Very low-calorie vegetables

Some green vegetables and salad leaves are so low in calories that you can serve your meal with a plate full of veg and still only add a few calories. Try squeezing over the juice of ½ lemon (2 cals) or dribbling over 1 teaspoon of balsamic vinegar (5 cals) to bring out the best in the flavour.

100g (3½oz/about ½ head) broccoli (33 cals)

100g (3½oz) green beans (24 cals)

100g (3½oz) mangetout (snow peas) (32 cals)

50g (1¾oz) baby spinach (12 cals)/watercress (11 cals)/rocket (arugula) (17 cals)

80g (3oz) bag mixed leaf salad (10–20 cals – check the packet to confirm)

Menu Plans for Diet Days

Plan A: Original 500 Cals

WEEK 1: 500 CALS				
	Breakfast	**Lunch**	**Dinner**	**Cals**
Day 1	Small banana 84 cals	Spicy Sweet Potato Soup 125 cals (page 91)	Baked Salmon & Asparagus 271 cals (page 114)	**480**
Day 2	Greek yogurt with berries 129 cals (page 51)	Spicy Sweet Potato Soup 125 cals (page 91)	Chicken Satay 244 cals (page 113)	**498**

WEEK 2: 500 CALS				
	Breakfast	**Lunch**	**Dinner**	**Cals**
Day 1	Fruity Bran Loaf 156 cals (page 54)	Carrot & Coriander Soup 116 cals (page 90)	Zesty Pork Steaks 224 cals (page 142)	**496**
Day 2	Fruity Bran Loaf 156 cals (page 54)	Carrot & Coriander Soup 116 cals (page 90)	Leek & Olive Pasta 233 cals (page 171)	**505**

WEEK 3: 500 CALS				
	Breakfast	**Lunch**	**Dinner**	**Cals**
Day 1	100g Natural Yogurt + 1/2 tsp honey 105 cals	Harissa Spiced Chickpeas 184 cals (page 69)	Coriander & Lemon Chicken 199 cals (page 110)	**488**
Day 2	Greek Yogurt with Berries 129 cals (page 51)	Harissa Spiced Chickpeas 184 cals (page 69)	Tiger Prawns with Aioli 167 cals (page 109)	**480**

WEEK 4: 500 CALS			
	Breakfast	Lunch	Dinner	Cals
Day 1	Small banana 84 cals	Mushroom & White Wine Soup 115 cals (page 89)	Salade Nicoise 300 cals (page 85)	**499**
Day 2	100g Natural Yogurt + 1/2 tsp honey 105 cals	Mushroom & White Wine Soup 115 cals (page 89)	Asian-style Beef & Mushrooms 267 cals (page 144)	**487**

Plan B: 800 Cals (Fast before)

WEEK 1: 800 CALS (FAST BEFORE)		
	Late Breakfast/Early Lunch	Dinner	Cals
Day 1	All-in-one Breakfast 270 cals (page 58)	Chicken Tikka Masala 456 cals (page 137)	**726**
Day 2	2 Ingredient Banana Pancakes 315 cals (page 64)	Shepherds Pie 479 cals (page 167)	**794**

WEEK 2: 800 CALS (FAST BEFORE)		
	Late Breakfast/Early Lunch	Dinner	Cals
Day 1	Mexican Five Bean Wrap 288 cals (page 80)	Turkey Meatballs in Tomato Sauce 452 cals (page 134)	**740**
Day 2	Fragrant Chicken 333 cals (page 117)	Pork Stir-fry with Noodles 417 cals (page 166)	**750**

WEEK 3: 800 CALS (FAST BEFORE)

	Late Breakfast/Early Lunch	Dinner	Cals
Day 1	Veggie Scrambled Eggs 298 cals (page 63)	Thai Chicken Curry 449 cals (page 132)	**747**
Day 2	Overnight Oats 294 cals (page 61)	Sweet & Sour Pork 493 cals (page 163)	**787**

WEEK 4: 800 CALS (FAST BEFORE)

	Late Breakfast/Early Lunch	Dinner	Cals
Day 1	Minestrone 276 cals (page 105)	Chicken & Broccoli in White Wine 456 cals (page 131)	**732**
Day 2	Chicken Salad Lemon Pepper Dressing 294 cals (page 82)	Sausage Cassoulet 413 cals (page 165)	**707**

Plan C: 800 Cals (Fast after)

WEEK 1: 800 CALS (FAST AFTER)

	Breakfast	Lunch	Early Dinner	Cals
Day 1	Small banana 84 cals	Savoy Cabbage & Bacon Soup 222 cals (page 99)	Steamed Salmon with Spicy Rice 468 cals (page 139)	**774**
Day 2	Greek yogurt with berries 129 cals (page 51)	Savoy Cabbage & Bacon Soup 222 cals (page 99)	Tomato Chicken Spaghetti 434 cals (page 128)	**785**

WEEK 2: 800 CALS (FAST AFTER)

	Breakfast	Lunch	Early Dinner	Cals
Day 1	Fruity Bran Loaf 156 cals (page 54)	Pear Salad with Roquefort 240 cals (page 70)	Beef with Mustard Sauce 401 cals (page 159)	**797**
Day 2	1/2 Grapefruit with 1/2 tsp sugar 49 cals	Greek Salad 265 cals (page 72)	Shepherds Pie 479 cals (page 167)	**793**

WEEK 3: 800 CALS (FAST AFTER)

	Breakfast	Lunch	Early Dinner	Cals
Day 1	Blueberry Muffin 142 cals (page 52)	Hearty Ham Soup 256 cals (page 103)	Chicken, Rice and Peas 399 cals (page 123)	**797**
Day 2	Blueberry Muffin 142 cals (page 52)	Hearty Ham Soup 256 cals (page 103)	Slow-cooked Chilli Beef Stew 401 cals (page 161)	**799**

WEEK 4: 800 CALS (FAST AFTER)

	Breakfast	Lunch	Early Dinner	Cals
Day 1	Fruity Bran Loaf 156 cals (page 54)	Fresh Garden Soup 169 cals (page 97)	Beef Burger with Sweet Potato Wedges 353 cals (page 155)	**678**
Day 2	Fruity Bran Loaf 156 cals (page 54)	Fresh Garden Soup 169 cals (page 97)	Egg-fried Rice with Prawns 432 cals (page 127)	**757**

The Recipes

This is a book of ideas for eating healthy, well-balanced and low calorie food, perfect for the days when you have to watch your calories.

Every recipe is designed to keep you feeling satisfied for longer. This is done by choosing lean proteins, low fats and complex carbohydrates and combining them with bold flavours. Although a few recipes require a smaller portion size, most provide you with a healthy 'normal' plate of food.

Some of the recipes are for one portion but could be doubled if required. Where this isn't practical, the recipe makes two servings, suitable for sharing or keeping for another day. There are also plenty of recipes suitable for serving to a larger group of people or dividing into portions and freezing. You can then have a portion ready when you get home from work with a minimal amount of fuss.

Finally, everything is simple to prepare and cook. The ingredients are all readily available in any supermarket. There's nothing too fancy or expensive here.

So please use this as an inspiration and a starting point for your own 5:2 cooking. Just because you're on a diet (for one day!) doesn't mean you have to be hungry...

Breakfast/Brunch

Greek Yogurt With Berries - 129 cals

Blueberry Muffins - 142 cals

Strawberry Smoothie - 147 cals

Fruity Bran Loaf - 156 cals

Nutty Banana Energy Bars - 242 cals

Baked Eggs With Ham And Tomato - 251 cals

All-in-one Breakfast - 270 cals

Continental Plate - 272 cals

Proper Porridge - 273 cals

Overnight Oats - 294 cals

Breakfast Burrito - 297 cals

Veggie Scrambled Eggs - 298 cals

2 Ingredient Banana Pancakes - 315 cals

Banana Slice - 303 cals

Greek Yogurt With Berries

129 calories

Serves 1 • Ready in 1 minute

100g (1/3 cup) Greek yogurt (96 cals)

1 tsp runny honey (23 cals)

handful fresh or frozen berries
(30g/1oz) (10 cals)

- Mix the greek yogurt and honey together. Sprinkle the berries over the top.

Blueberry Muffins

142 calories

Makes 10 muffins • Ready in 30 minutes

150g (generous 1 cup) plain
(all-purpose) flour (512 cals)
....
100g (¾ cup) self-raising
(self-rising) flour (330 cals)
....
1 tbsp oat bran (25 cals)
....
2 tsp baking powder (14 cals)
....
½ tsp bicarbonate of soda (baking soda)
....
pinch of salt
....
50g (¼ cup) muscovado (soft
brown) sugar (181 cals)
....
200ml (generous ¾ cup)
buttermilk (94 cals)
....
1 tbsp runny honey (86 cals)
....
1 large egg (91 cals)
....
150g (1 cup) fresh blueberries (86 cals)
....

- Preheat the oven to 180C/160C fan/350F. Line a muffin tray with 10 paper cases.

- Mix all the dry ingredients together in a large bowl. Whisk the honey and egg into the buttermilk with a fork.

- Pour the wet ingredients over the dry and mix until well combined. Don't worry if the mix is still a little lumpy, it is better to under rather than overmix. Fold in the blueberries.

- Spoon the batter into the paper cases and bake in the oven for 20-25 minutes, until turning brown on the top.

Strawberry Smoothie

147 calories

Serves 1 • Ready in 5 minutes

5 strawberries, hulled (20 cals)

½ banana (53 cals)

1 tbsp fat-free greek yogurt (10 cals)

200ml (generous ¾ cup)
skimmed milk (64 cals)

- This is a simple one. Place all the ingredients in a blender and whizz until smooth. Serve immediately.

Fruity Bran Loaf

156 calories (per slice)

Makes 10 slices • Ready in 45 minutes (plus 30 minutes rest)

100g (1½ cups) All-Bran (or similar,
but not bran flakes) (270 cals)

....

90g (½ cup) caster (superfine)
sugar (355 cals)

....

100g (½ cup) sultanas (golden
raisins) (275 cals)

....

50g (¼ cup) dried apricots,
chopped (94 cals)

....

50g (1¾oz) dried figs, chopped (114 cals)

....

50g (1¾oz) dates, chopped (62 cals)

....

250ml (generous 1 cup) skimmed
(skim) milk (80 cals)

....

light oil spray (3 cals)

....

100g (¾ cup) wholemeal self-raising
(wholewheat self-rising) flour (310 cals)

....

- Put the All-Bran, sugar and dried fruit into a bowl and mix together well. Stir in the milk and leave to stand for 30 minutes.

- Preheat the oven to 180C/160C fan/350F and oil a loaf tin (pan) well with oil spray.

- Sift in the flour, mixing well. Pour the mixture into the prepared loaf tin (loaf pan) and bake for 35–40 minutes. Turn out of the tin immediately and leave to cool on a wire rack.

-

Nutty Banana Energy Bars

242 calories each

Makes 8 bars • Ready in 1 hour

light oil spray (3 cals)
50g (¼ cup) quinoa, well rinsed (154 cals)
170g (2 cups) porridge (rolled) oats (605 cals)
1 tsp ground cinnamon
1 tsp baking powder (7 cals)
2 tbsp desiccated (dry unsweetened) coconut (98 cals)
pinch of salt
50g ($1/^3$ cup) dried cranberries (162 cals)
30g (¼ cup) pecans, chopped (207 cals)
3 medium very ripe bananas, mashed (356 cals)
1 large egg, beaten (91 cals)
50g (4 tbsp) maple syrup (131 cals)
1 tbsp sunflower oil (99 cals)
2 tsp vanilla extract (24 cals)

- Line a 25 × 25cm (10 × 10in) baking tray (cookie sheet) with two pieces of baking parchment, forming a cross shape so that all the sides are covered and spray with light oil spray.

- Place the quinoa and 125ml (½ cup) water in a small saucepan and bring to the boil. Reduce the heat and simmer gently for 12–15 minutes or until the liquid is just absorbed. Remove from the heat and rest, covered, for 5 minutes. Transfer to a bowl and fluff with a fork. Leave to cool completely.

- Preheat the oven to 160C/140C fan/325F.

- Place the oats, cinnamon, baking powder, desiccated coconut and salt in a large bowl and mix thoroughly. Then mix in the dried cranberries and chopped pecans.
- Add the mashed bananas, beaten egg, maple syrup, oil and vanilla to the quinoa and stir until just combined. Add the banana mixture to the oat mixture and loosely mix.
- Press the batter into the prepared baking tray and bake in the oven for 35–40 minutes. Leave to cool completely in the tray.
- When cool, lift out using the baking parchment and transfer to a chopping board. Cut into 8 bars. Wrap individually in clingfilm (plastic wrap) and store in the refrigerator for up to a week. Alternatively, store in an airtight container in the freezer for up to three months.

Baked Eggs With Ham And Tomato

251 calories

Serves 1 • Ready in 15 minutes

½ leek, trimmed and thinly sliced (13 cals)

½ tsp olive oil (14 cals)

1 slice ham, chopped (41 cals)

1 large egg (91 cals)

2 slices tomato (9 cals)

20g (scant ¼ cup) Cheddar
cheese, grated (83 cals)

- Preheat the oven to 180C/160C fan/350F.
- Place the leek and oil in a small microwaveable dish. Cover with clingfilm (plastic wrap) and microwave on high for 4 minutes. Leave to rest, still covered, for a further 2 minutes.
- Place the leek at the bottom of a ramekin and top with the ham.
- Pour in the egg, then top with the tomato slices and sprinkle with the cheese.
- Bake in the oven for 10 minutes or until the egg is set and the top is turning brown.

All-in-one Breakfast

270 calories

Serves 1 • Ready in 15 minutes

1 good-quality sausage (50g/1¾oz),
sliced (154 calories)
....
100g (3½oz) mushrooms, sliced (13 cals)
....
1 medium tomato, roughly
chopped (14 cals)
....
1 large egg, beaten (89 cals)
....

- Put your frying pan (skillet) over a medium heat. When hot, add the sausage and cook, turning every 1–2 minutes, for 8 minutes until browned on all sides.

- Add the mushrooms to the pan and fry in the sausage fat for about 3 minutes until browned. Push your mushrooms and sausage to the side, add the tomato and fry for 2 minutes.

- Pour the egg into the pan and stir into the tomato. Fry slowly, stirring often, until scrambled but still soft. Serve immediately.

Continental Plate

272 calories

Serves 1 • Ready in 10 minutes

1 large egg (91 cals)

....

2 crisp lettuce leaves, such as
Little Gem/Boston (2 cals)

....

1 tomato, quartered (14 cals)

....

1 chunky slice of good-quality
ham, cut into 4 pieces (36 cals)

....

2 thick slices (30g/1oz)
Gouda cheese (129 cals)

....

- First lightly boil your egg by placing it gently into a pan of simmering water. Cook for 7–9 minutes, depending on how you like it cooked. Remove from the pan with a slotted spoon and cool for a few minutes before peeling and cutting into quarters.

- Arrange the lettuce and tomatoes over one side of the plate, with the ham and cheese arranged on the other side. Finally place the quartered egg in the centre.

Proper Porridge

273 cals

Serves 1 • Ready in 5 minutes

40g (1½ oz) porridge (rolled) oats (143 cals)
....
200ml (1 cup) semi-skimmed milk (98 cals)
....
1 heaped tsp dark brown sugar (32 cals)
....

- Place the oats and milk in a saucepan and heat on the hob. As soon as the milk gets hot, start to stir and stir continuously until the porridge has a creamy consistency. Depending on the thickness you like, this could be anything from 2 to 5 minutes. Serve with the brown sugar sprinkled over.

Overnight Oats

294 calories

Serves 1 • Ready in 5 minutes, plus overnight resting (optional)

40g (1½oz) porridge oats
(rolled) oats (143 cals)
....
150ml (²/³ cup) semi-skimmed
milk (74 cals)
....
1 tbsp natural plain yogurt (22 cals)
....
10g toasted flaked almonds (62 cals)
....
1 tsp runny honey (23 cals)
....

• Simply place all your ingredients in a bowl or jar with a screw-top lid. If it's a bowl, stir thoroughly. If it's a jar, put the lid on and shake vigorously. You can rest the oats for as long or as little as you prefer.

Breakfast Burrito

297 calories

Serves 1 • Ready in 5 minutes

1 slice (15g/½oz) streaky
bacon, chopped (50 cals)
....
½ green (bell) pepper (12 cals)
....
2 spring onions (scallions),
chopped (10 cals)
....
1 large egg, beaten (89 cals)
....
1 soft tortilla wrap (125 cals)
....
1 tsp salsa (4 cals)
....
1 tsp natural yogurt (7 cals)
....

- Fry the bacon, pepper and spring onions (scallions) together for about 5 minutes.

- Add the beaten egg and scramble until just set.

- Heat the tortilla for 10 seconds on a plate in the microwave. Fill with scrambled egg and top with the salsa and yogurt, tuck in the ends, and roll up!

Veggie Scrambled Eggs

298 calories per serving

Serves 1 • Ready in 10 mins

1 tsp olive oil (27 cals)
....
½ onion, finely diced (27 cals)
....
1 clove garlic, sliced (4 cals)
....
½ green (bell) pepper, de-seeded
and diced (12 cals)
....
2 large tomatoes, chopped (36 cals)
....
1 tsp tomato paste (10 cals)
....
2 tbsp water
....
2 large eggs (182 cals)
....
3 fresh basil leaves if you have them
....

- Heat the oil in a frying pan and add the onions, garlic and peppers. Fry them gently on a medium heat for 5 minutes, until golden. Add in the tomatoes, tomato paste and water and cook for another 2 minutes.

- Meanwhile, whisk the eggs together and season with salt and pepper. Pour the eggs into the frying pan with the other ingredients, stirring constantly until they thicken like scrambled eggs – about 3 minutes. Serve with basil on the top.

2 Ingredient Banana Pancakes

315 calories

Serves 1 • Ready in 10 minutes

1 banana (106 cals)

....

2 eggs (182 cals)

....

1 tsp mild olive oil (27 cals)

....

- Use the back of a fork to thoroughly mash the banana.

- In a separate bowl, whisk the eggs. Add the banana to the whisked eggs.

- Heat the oil in a medium frying pan until hot but not smoking. Pour in the pancake mix. Cook for 3-4 minutes, turning if you dare until just cooked but still a little wobbly.

Banana Slice

303 calories

Makes 10 slices • Ready in 1hr 15 mins

1 tbsp chia seeds (84 cals)
....
3 medium ripe bananas (330g) (357 cals)
....
1 tsp vanilla essence (12 cals)
....
3 tbsp mild olive oil (297 cals)
....
50g (¼ cup) caster (superfine)
sugar (197 cals)
....
50g (¼ cup) demerara (raw
brown) sugar (197 cals)
....
2 tbsp runny honey (60g/2oz) (173 cals)
....
1 tsp baking powder
....
½ tsp salt
....
½ tsp ground cinnamon
....
180ml (¾ cup) skimmed
(skim) milk (67 cals)
....
100g (1 cup) almond flour (613 cals)
....
200g (1¼ cup) wholemeal (wholewheat
self-rising) self-raising flour (620 cals)
....
110g (1¼ cup) jumbo oats (411 cals)
....

- Place the chia seeds in a small bowl or cup. Add 2 1/2 tbsp water and leave for 5 minutes to absorb.

- Preheat the oven to 190C/170C fan/350F. Line a large (9x5 inch) loaf tin (pan) with greaseproof (parchment) paper.

- Mash the bananas in a large bowl. Add the vanilla, olive oil, caster (superfine) sugar, demerara (raw brown) sugar and honey. Mix well.

- Next add the baking powder, salt, cinnamon, soaked chia and milk. Stir again. Don't worry if it looks like a brown sticky mess at this stage!

- Finally add the almond flour, self-raising flour and oats and stir.
- Transfer to the loaf tin (pan) and bake for 1 hour to 1 hour 15 minutes. When cooked, it will feel firm to the touch and golden brown on the top.
- Cool completely before cutting. Will store in an airtight container for 3 days. Can be frozen in individual slices.

Light Lunch

Harissa Spiced Chickpeas - 184 cals

Pear Salad With Roquefort - 240 cals

Warm Courgette And Mozzarella Salad - 263 cals

Greek Salad - 265 cals

Warm Puy Lentil & Goat's Cheese Salad - 272 cals

Avocado And Bacon Salad - 274 cals

Quinoa With Red Peppers And Broccoli - 278 cals

North African Chicken Salad - 279 cals

Asian Chicken Salad - 285 cals

Stuffed Avocado - 284 cals

Mexican Five Bean Wrap - 288 cals

Tuna And Bean Salad - 289 cals

Chicken Salad & Lemon Pepper Dressing - 294 cals

Bulgur Wheat Lunchbox Salad - 295 cals

Chilli Chicken Pitta - 298 cals

Salade Nicoise - 300 cals

Harissa Spiced Chickpeas

184 calories

Serves 2 • Ready in 10 minutes

1 tbsp harissa paste (13 cals)

1 tbsp tomato purée (paste) (30 cals)

1 × 400g (14oz) can chickpeas,
rinsed and drained (276 cals)

juice of ½ lemon (2 cals)

200g (7oz) fresh green beans,
trimmed (48 cals)

- Heat the harissa and tomato purée (paste) in a frying pan (skillet) over a medium heat for 1–2 minutes, until it just starts to sizzle. Reduce the heat to low and stir in the chickpeas and lemon juice. Cook for 2–3 minutes, until warmed through.

- Cook the green beans in a pan of boiling water until just tender, about 4 minutes.

- Serve the chickpeas over the green beans.

Pear Salad With Roquefort

240 calories

Serves 1 • Ready in 5 minutes

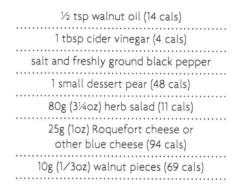

½ tsp walnut oil (14 cals)

1 tbsp cider vinegar (4 cals)

salt and freshly ground black pepper

1 small dessert pear (48 cals)

80g (3¼oz) herb salad (11 cals)

25g (1oz) Roquefort cheese or
other blue cheese (94 cals)

10g (1/3oz) walnut pieces (69 cals)

- Mix the walnut oil, vinegar and a little salt and pepper together to make a dressing.

- Cut the pear into quarters, remove the cores and cut each quarter into 4 slices.

- Arrange the herb salad on a serving plate and arrange the pear attractively over it. Crumble the cheese over the top, followed by the walnuts. Pour over the dressing and eat straight away.

Warm Courgette And Mozzarella Salad

263 calories

Serves 1 • Ready in 10 minutes

1 large or 2 small courgettes (zucchini)
(250g/9oz), trimmed (45 cals)

20 cherry tomatoes, quartered (45 cals)

zest of ½ lemon (1 cal)

1 tbsp balsamic vinegar (12 cals)

1 tsp extra virgin olive oil (27 cals)

½ tsp olive oil (13 cals)

½ garlic clove, peeled and crushed (or
½ tsp garlic purée/paste) (2 cals)

salt and freshly ground black pepper

5 fresh basil leaves

½ ball light Italian mozzarella
(75 g) (119 cals)

- Use a vegetable peeler or mandoline to cut your courgette (zucchini) into ribbons. Discard the first slice as it will be mainly skin. If using the vegetable peeler, make slices until you hit the seeds, then rotate and peel again. Press the courgette (zucchini) between two sheets of kitchen paper to absorb excess moisture.

- Mix the tomatoes, lemon zest, balsamic vinegar and extra virgin olive oil together in a bowl.

- In a wide frying pan (skillet), heat the olive oil over a medium-high heat. When hot, toss in the garlic and fry for 1 minute. Add the courgette, then season with salt and pepper and cook for 2 minutes. Give it a stir and cook for a further 1–2 minutes or until the courgette is cooked through yet firm.

- Transfer the courgette to a serving bowl and pour the tomato mixture over. Tear the basil and mozzarella and place on top.

Greek Salad

265 calories

Serves 1 • Ready in 5 minutes

1 tsp extra virgin olive oil (27 cals)
....

1 tsp white wine vinegar (1 cal)
....

pinch of sugar (4 cals)
....

salt and freshly ground black pepper
....

2 fresh basil leaves, finely chopped
....

1 × 80g (3oz) bag mixed leaf salad (16 cals)
....

5cm (2in) piece cucumber,
roughly diced (10 cals)
....

2 medium tomatoes, roughly
diced (28 cals)
....

2 spring onions (scallions), trimmed
and shredded (10 cals)
....

50g (1¾oz) feta cheese, cut
into small cubes (138 cals)
....

6 black olives, pitted (31 cals)
....

- In a small bowl, stir together the olive oil, vinegar, sugar, salt and pepper and basil leaves.

- Put the salad leaves in a wide bowl or container and lightly toss in the cucumber, tomatoes and spring onions (scallions). Drizzle over the dressing and toss again.

- Arrange the feta and black olives over the top and serve.

Warm Puy Lentil And Goat's Cheese Salad

272 calories

You can also use ready-to-eat lentils to make this salad super quick.

Serves 1 • Ready in 30 minutes

40g (1½oz) dried Puy (French green) lentils (119 cals)
....
15 cherry tomatoes (34 cals)
....
50g (1¾oz) baby spinach leaves (12 cals)
....
30g (1¼oz) pickled sweet peppers in brine, drained and roughly chopped (33 cals)
....
2 fresh basil leaves, shredded
....
1 tbsp balsamic vinegar (14 cals)
....
salt and freshly ground black pepper
....
30g (1¼oz) goat's cheese (60 cals)
....

- Cook the Puy lentils in a pan of boiling water for about 25 minutes, or according to the packet instructions. Leave the lentils to cool slightly; they are perfect warm but not hot.

- When the lentils are warm, combine them with the cherry tomatoes, baby spinach, sweet peppers and basil leaves in a large bowl. Pour the balsamic vinegar over, season with a little salt and pepper and toss well.

- Transfer to a serving dish, crumble the goat's cheese over the top and serve while still warm.

Avocado And Bacon Salad

274 calories

Serves 1 • Ready in 10 minutes

15g (½oz) streaky bacon, chopped
(about 1 slice) (50 cals)
....
¼ red onion, finely sliced (14 cals)
....
½ red (bell) pepper, finely sliced (26 cals)
....
1 × 80g (3oz) bag mixed leaf salad (16 cals)
....
½ ripe avocado, sliced (138 cals)
....
1 tsp extra virgin olive oil (27 cals)
....
juice of ¼ lemon (1 cal)
....
salt and freshly ground black pepper
....

- Heat a small frying pan (skillet) over a medium–high heat and fry the bacon until brown and crisp. Dry and cool on kitchen paper (paper towels).

- Using the oil left in the pan from the bacon, reduce the heat a little and fry the onion and red (bell) pepper for 5–7 minutes until tender and golden.

- Place the salad leaves in a wide bowl and mix through the onion and red pepper. Add the sliced avocado and drizzle with the olive oil and lemon juice. Season with salt and pepper and top with the crispy bacon.

Quinoa With Red Peppers And Broccoli

278 calories

Serves 1 • Ready in 10 minutes

1 red (bell) pepper, de-seeded and
cut into long strips (54 cals)

....

50g (¼ cup) dried quinoa,
well rinsed (154 cals)

....

100g (3½oz) broccoli, cut
into florets (33 cals)

....

1 tsp olive oil (27 cals)

....

1 shallot, finely diced (6 cals)

....

1 garlic clove, finely sliced (4 cals)

....

1 bay leaf

....

½ tsp dried oregano

....

Small handful fresh parsley, chopped

....

Small handful fresh coriander, chopped

....

- Put the pepper strips on a grill tray and grill on a medium heat for about 10 minutes, turning once, until tender and black at the edges.

- Rinse the quinoa before placing in a saucepan along with the broccoli. Add the bay leaf and oregano. Add 250ml water and simmer gently until the water is absorbed – about 8 minutes.

- In a shallow pan heat the oil gently and fry the shallots and garlic for 10 minutes.

- Stir the peppers, shallots and herbs into the quinoa. Season with salt and pepper.

North African Chicken Salad

279 calories

Serves 2 • Ready in 10 minutes

10cm (4 in) cucumber, cubed (20 cals)

10 cherry tomatoes, halved (22 cals)

½ red (bell) pepper, seeded
and diced (26 cals)

2 spring onions (scallions),
finely chopped (9 cals)

1 tbsp sultanas (golden raisins) (54 cals)

4 parsley leaves, shredded

2 Little Gem (Boston) lettuces,
shredded (44 cals)

1 x 125g (4oz) roasted cooked chicken
breast, skin removed (178 cals)

1 tbsp toasted pine nuts (138 cals)

For the dressing:

2 tsp extra virgin olive oil (54 cals)

Zest and juice of ½ orange (11 cals)

½ clove garlic, finely chopped (2 cals)

1 tsp ground cumin

½ tsp brown sugar

salt and pepper

- Mix together the dressing ingredients in a small cup or bowl and set aside to rest for 5 minutes.

- Place the cucumber, tomatoes, red pepper, spring onions (scallions), lettuce and parsley in another large bowl and toss the dressing over, making sure everything is well-coated.

- Divide the salad between 2 plates and arrange the chicken and toasted pine nuts over the top.

Asian Chicken Salad

285 calories

Serves 2 • Ready in 35 minutes

250g (19oz) skinless, boneless chicken
breast, cut into strips (370 cals)

½ onion, peeled and roughly
chopped (27 cals)

1 bay leaf

1 stalk lemongrass, bruised
with the back of a knife

For the salad:

½ cucumber, peeled (20 cals)

a pinch of salt

1 celery stick, cut into long,
thin strips (5 cals)

1 medium carrot, peeled and cut
into long, thin strips (35 cals)

80g (3¼oz) white cabbage,
thinly shredded (22 cals)

1 small handful of fresh coriander
(cilantro) leaves, roughly chopped (3 cals)

1 small handful of fresh mint leaves,
roughly chopped (6 cals)

2 tsp sesame seeds (60 cals)

6 Little Gem (Boston) lettuce
leaves, shredded (3 cals)

For the dressing:

½ garlic clove, peeled and crushed (2 cals)

½ small red chilli, deseeded
and cut into rings (1 cal)

½ tsp granulated sugar (10 cals)

juice of 1 lime (4 cals)

....

1 tsp fish sauce (1 cal)

....

salt and freshly ground black pepper

....

- Place the chicken in a lidded saucepan and add the onion, bay leaf and lemongrass. Cover with water and bring to the boil. Put the lid on the pan, reduce the heat and simmer for 10–12 minutes or until the chicken is cooked. Remove the chicken from the pan with a slotted spoon and leave to cool.

- For the salad, using a vegetable peeler, cut the cucumber into flat strips. Place between 2 sheets of kitchen paper to absorb some of the water. Leave for a few minutes.

- Meanwhile, make the dressing by placing all the dressing ingredients in a small bowl, adding 1 tablespoon water and mixing together.

- Place the cucumber in a large bowl and add the celery, carrot, cabbage and herbs. Mix in the cooked chicken and half the sesame seeds, then stir in the dressing.

- Arrange the lettuce leaves on 2 serving plates, then pile the salad on top of the lettuce and sprinkle with the remaining sesame seeds. Serve.

Stuffed Avocado

284 calories

Serves 1 • Ready in 5 minutes

1 medium ripe avocado (250 cals)

6 cherry tomatoes, cut into
quarters (14 cals)

100g (3½oz) cucumber
(5cm/2in piece), peeled

and cut into small cubes (10 cals)

2 tsp good-quality balsamic
vinegar (10 cals)

salt and freshly ground black pepper

- Prepare the avocado by cutting it in half and removing the stone (pit). Mix the tomatoes, cucumber and vinegar together in a small bowl, then season with salt and pepper and spoon over the avocados. Serve immediately.

Mexican Five Bean Wrap

288 calories

Serves 1 • Ready in 3 minutes

1 soft tortilla wrap (125 cals)
....
80g (3oz) ready-to-eat mixed
beans, drained (81 cals)
....
15g (½oz) cheddar, grated (62 cals)
....
1 tbsp salsa (13 cals)
....
shredded lettuce (7 cals)
....

• Rinse and drain the beans. Spread the salsa evenly over the
  whole wrap. Then add the beans, making sure you leave at least
  an inch free at the bottom of the wrap to fold over. Arrange
  your shredded lettuce over the beans and then grate over the
  cheese as evenly as possible. Fold over the bottom inch of the
  wrap. Then gently but firmly roll up the wrap.

Tuna And Bean Salad

289 calories

Serves 1 • Ready in 15 minutes

¼ red onion, peeled and
finely chopped (16 cals)

juice of 1 lemon (4 cals)

½ × 400g (14oz) can mixed beans,
rinsed and drained (134 cals)

1 × 160g (7oz) can good-quality
tuna in water, drained (111 cals)

5cm (2in) piece cucumber, cut
into small chunks (10 cals)

1 small handful of fresh flat-leaf
(Italian) parsley leaves, chopped

½ tsp extra-virgin olive oil (14 cals)

salt and freshly ground black pepper

- Put the chopped onion into a bowl and stir in the lemon juice. Cover with clingfilm (plastic wrap) and microwave for 1 minute. Leave to cool.

- Place the drained beans in a wide bowl and flake the tuna into the beans. Add the cucumber and stir through the chopped parsley.

- Add the olive oil to the onions and season with salt and pepper, then pour the onion mixture over the tuna and beans. Stir through and leave at room temperature for another 10 minutes to allow the flavours to fully develop before serving.

Chicken Salad With Lemon Pepper Dressing

294 calories

Serves 1 • Ready in 5 minutes

1 tbsp low-fat crème fraîche (57 cals)
juice of ½ lemon (2 cals)
freshly ground black pepper
pinch of salt
pinch of sugar (4 cals)
1 × 80g (3oz) bag baby leaf or herb salad (16 cals)
5cm (2in) piece cucumber, finely sliced (10 cals)
1 medium tomato, sliced (14 cals)
1 cooked chicken breast (125g/4oz) (191 cals)

- Combine the crème fraîche, lemon juice, black pepper, salt and sugar in a small bowl.

- Arrange the salad leaves, cucumber and tomato in a wide bowl.

- Cut the chicken into thick slices and arrange on top of the salad. Drizzle the dressing over and serve.

Bulgur Wheat Lunchbox Salad

295 calories

Serves 1 • Ready in 20 minutes

50g (¹/³ cup) cracked bulgur
wheat (176 cals)

salt and freshly ground black pepper

50g (1¾oz) frozen broad
(fava) beans (30 cals)

4 radishes, thinly sliced (4 cals)

¼ red onion, peeled and very
thinly sliced (14 cals)

small handful of fresh mint,
chopped (10 g) (4 cals)

zest and juice of 1 lime (4 cals)

½ small red chilli, deseeded
and finely chopped (2 cals)

1 tsp extra virgin olive oil (27 cals)

1 tsp white wine vinegar (1 cal)

½ tsp English mustard (6 cal)

1 tsp runny honey (23 cals)

- Place the bulgur wheat in a bowl and season with salt and pepper. Pour on 100ml (scant ½ cup) just boiled water, then cover and leave to cook for 15 minutes until tender.

- Cook the broad (fava) beans in boiling water for 4–5 minutes, then combine the broad beans with the bulgur wheat and leave to cool. When the beans and bulgur wheat are cool, stir through the radishes, red onion and mint.

- In a small bowl, mix together the lime zest and juice, chilli, olive oil, vinegar, mustard and honey. Pour over the salad, then serve immediately or cover and keep refrigerated until needed.

Chilli Chicken Pitta

298 calories

Serves 1 • Ready in 15 minutes

1 spring onion (scallion),
chopped finely (5 cals)
....
½ garlic clove, chopped finely (2 cals)
....
juice ½ lime (2 cals)
....
½ tsp runny honey (12 cals)
....
¼ tsp paprika (4 cals)
....
¼ tsp mild chilli powder
....
100g (3½oz) cooked chicken breast fillet,
chopped into really small pieces (113 cals)
....
1 pitta bread (154 cals)
....
A little iceberg lettuce, shredded (7 cals)
....

- Mix together the spring onion (scallion), garlic, lime juice, honey, paprika and chilli powder. Stir the chicken into the marinade. Leave to rest for 5 minutes.

- Toast your pitta lightly. Cut in half and stuff with the shredded lettuce and dressed chicken.

Salade Nicoise

300 calories

Serves 1 • Ready in 5 minutes

1 Little Gem (Boston) lettuce,
separated into leaves (17 cals)
....
1 tomato, quartered (14 cals)
....
1 hard-boiled egg, cut into
quarters (90 cals)
....
40g (1½oz) green beans, cooked
(from fresh or frozen) (10 cals)
....
100g (4oz) canned tuna in
water or brine (113 cals)
....
5 black olives (26 cals)
....
For the dressing:
....
1 tsp extra virgin olive oil (27 cals)
....
1 tsp cider vinegar (1 cal)
....
1 tsp capers (2 cals)
....
salt and pepper
....

- Mix together the dressing ingredients and set aside. Place the
lettuce leaves in a bowl and add the tomato, green beans and
hard-boiled egg. Roughly flake the tuna and add in. Pour the
dressing over the salad. Top with the anchovy fillet and scatter
over the olives.

Soups

Creamy Mushroom & White Wine Soup -115 cals

Carrot And Coriander Soup -116 cals

Spicy Sweet Potato Soup -125 cals

Borscht (Chunky Beetroot Soup) -134 cals

Roasted Parsnip Soup -139 cals

Slow Onion Soup -197 cals

Mexican Chicken Soup -162 cals

Fresh Garden Soup -169 cals

Savoy Cabbage And Bacon Soup -222 cals

Butternut Soup With Goat's Cheese -226 cals

Chorizo And Tomato Soup -233 cals

Lentil, Lemon And Thyme Soup -233 cals

Hearty Ham Soup -256 cals

Spicy Ramen With Rice Noodles -258 cals

Minestrone -276 cals

Creamy Mushroom And White Wine Soup

115 calories

Serves 4 • Ready in 40 minutes

1 tsp olive oil (27 cals)
....
1 large onion, peeled and
finely chopped (86 cals)
....
1 garlic clove, finely sliced (3 cals)
....
400g (14oz) mushrooms, sliced (52 cals)
....
1¼ litres (5 cups) vegetable stock (fresh
or made with 2 cubes) (70 cals)
....
1 bay leaf
....
10g (2 tsp) butter (74 cals)
....
200ml (generous ¾ cup)
white wine (66 cals)
....
50g (3 tbsp/¼ cup) light
soft cheese (78 cals)
....
handful of fresh parsley, chopped (3 cals)
....
salt and freshly ground black pepper
....

- Heat the oil in a large saucepan, add the onion and gently fry for 7 minutes. Add the garlic and fry for a further 2 minutes.

- Add about three-quarters of the mushrooms, turn in the oil then add the stock and bay leaf. Put a lid on and simmer for 15 minutes until the mushrooms are soft.

- Remove the bay leaf and blend until smooth.

- Heat the butter in a frying pan (skillet). When the butter has melted, toss in the remaining mushrooms and fry, turning once, until lightly browned.

- Return the blended soup to the pan and stir in the wine, cheese and parsley. Reheat gently and season to taste. Serve the soup with the fried mushrooms scattered on the top.

Carrot And Coriander Soup

116 calories

Serves 4 • Ready in 30 minutes

1 large onion, peeled and
chopped (86 cals)
....
500g (1lb 2oz) carrots, about
6 medium (175 cals)
....
1 small potato (100g/3 ½ oz),
peeled and chopped (75 cals)
....
1 tsp ground coriander
....
1 litre (4 cups) vegetable stock (fresh
or made with 2 cubes) (70 cals)
....
large handful of fresh coriander (cilantro)
....
freshly ground black pepper
....
4 tsp extra virgin olive oil (108 cals)
....

- Simply place the onion, carrots, potato and ground coriander in a large saucepan and pour in the stock. Bring to the boil, reduce the heat and simmer for 15-18 minutes until tender.

- Blitz in a blender or food processor with the fresh coriander until smooth. Return the soup to the pan and reheat gently.

- Serve with lashings of black pepper and a drizzle (1 teaspoon) of extra virgin olive oil.

Spicy Sweet Potato Soup

125 calories

Serves 2 • Ready in 30 minutes

1 tsp olive oil (27 cals)

2 small sweet potatoes, peeled
and roughly chopped (174 cals)

2 garlic cloves, peeled and crushed (6 cals)

1 tsp medium curry powder (7 cals)

½ tsp smoked paprika (3 cals)

1 tsp cornflour (cornstarch) (5 cals)

½ vegetable stock (bouillon) cube (17 cals)

1 tsp tomato ketchup (8 cals)

juice of 1 lemon (3 cals)

- Heat the oil in a saucepan, add the sweet potatoes and garlic and fry for 4–5 minutes. Sprinkle in the curry powder, paprika and cornflour (cornstarch) and stir-fry for 1 more minute.

- Add 2 tablespoons water and stir to form a paste (this is to stop the cornflour going lumpy) before adding 470ml (2 cups) water. Crumble in the stock (bouillon) cube and add the ketchup and lemon juice. Bring to the boil, then reduce the heat and simmer for 15–20 minutes or until the sweet potato is tender.

- Transfer to a blender and blend until smooth, then serve.

Borscht (Chunky Beetroot Soup)

134 calories

Serves 4 • Ready in 30 minutes

1 tbsp sunflower oil (99 cals)

1 carrot, peeled and chopped (35 cals)

1 medium onion, peeled
and chopped (54 cals)

1 celery stick, trimmed and
chopped (5 cals)

1 small parsnip (60g/2¼oz),
peeled and chopped (38 cals)

1 litre (4 cups) vegetable stock (fresh is
best but you could use 2 cubes) (70 cals)

500g (1lb 2oz) cooked beetroot (in natural
juice) chopped into large chunks (230 cals)

juice of ½ lemon (2 cals)

freshly ground black pepper

- Heat the oil in a large lidded saucepan over a low heat, add the carrot, onion, celery and parsnip, then stir and put the lid on. Allow the vegetables to sweat for 10 minutes.

- Add the stock, bring to the boil, then reduce the heat and simmer with the lid off for 10 minutes. Add the beetroot and simmer for another 5 minutes.

- Add the lemon juice and pepper to taste.

Roasted Parsnip Soup

139 calories

Serves 4 • Ready in 45 minutes

1 tbsp olive oil (99 cals)
6 medium parsnips (about 80g/3oz each), peeled and cut into large cubes (307 cals)
salt and freshly ground black pepper
1 tsp olive oil (27 cals)
1 small onion, peeled and finely chopped (22 cals)
zest of 1 lemon (2 cals)
¼ tsp vanilla extract
500ml (generous 2 cups) vegetable stock, fresh or from 1 cube (35 cals)
200ml (generous ¾ cup) skimmed (skim) milk (64 cals)

- Preheat the oven to 190C/170C fan/375F.

- Pour the 1 tablespoon olive oil over the parsnips and season generously with salt and pepper. Use your hands to toss the parsnips in the oil, making sure they are well covered.

- Spread the parsnips out over a baking tray and roast in the oven for 20 minutes.

- While the parsnips are in the oven, heat the 1 teaspoon oil in a large saucepan, add the onion and fry gently for 10 minutes until softened.

- Add the lemon zest, vanilla, stock and 100ml (scant ½ cup) water, then bring to the boil.

- Add the roasted parsnips and return to the boil. Reduce the heat, put the lid on and simmer gently for a further 15 minutes.

- Transfer to a blender and blend until smooth. Return to the pan, add the milk and stir. Reheat gently and serve.

Slow Onion Soup

197 calories

Serves 4 • Ready in 2 hours

1 tbsp olive oil (99 cals)
....
15g (1 tbsp) butter (112 cals)
....
1kg (2¼lb) onions, peeled and
finely sliced (360 cals)
....
1 garlic clove, peeled and
finely sliced (3 cals)
....
2 fresh thyme leaves, finely
chopped (or 1 tsp dried thyme)
....
1 bay leaf
....
salt and freshly ground black pepper
....
150ml (²/³ cup) red wine (129 cals)
....
1¼ litres (5 cups) beef stock (fresh is really
good here, but can use 2 cubes) (70 cals)
....
1 tsp caster sugar (16 cals)
....

- Heat the oil and butter gently in a wide lidded frying pan (skillet). When the butter has melted, add the onions, garlic, thyme and bay leaf. Season generously with salt and pepper and stir.

- With the heat on the lowest possible setting, put the lid on the pan and cook for about 1 hour, stirring occasionally.

- Add the wine, stock and sugar, then bring to the boil, reduce the heat and simmer for 30 minutes before serving.

Mexican Chicken Soup

162 calories

Serves 2 • Ready in 1 hour

2 chicken drumsticks (178 cals)
....
1 shallot, peeled and roughly
chopped (6 cals)
....
1 small carrot, peeled and
roughly chopped (28 cals)
....
1 stick celery, trimmed and
finely chopped (5 cals)
....
500ml (generous 2 cups) water
....
1x400g (14oz) can chopped
tomatoes (64 cals)
....
1 green (bell) pepper, deseeded
and chopped (24 cals)
....
1 clove garlic, peeled and crushed (4 cals)
....
1 tsp dried mixed herbs
....
½ tsp paprika (7 cals)
....
½ tsp smoked paprika (7 cals)
....
¼ tsp turmeric
....
¼ tsp ground cumin
....
1 tsp salt
....
Freshly ground black pepper
....
1 tsp mild chilli powder
....
Handful flat leaf (Italian) parsley,
stalks removed and chopped
....

- Place the chicken drumsticks, shallots, carrot and celery in a large saucepan. Pour over the water and bring up to a simmer. Cook for 20 minutes, then remove the chicken drumsticks with a slotted spoon and set aside to cool.

- Add the chopped tomatoes, green pepper and garlic and bring back up to simmering point. Add the dried herbs, paprika, smoked paprika, turmeric, cumin, salt, black pepper and chilli powder, then simmer gently for 30 minutes.

- Remove the skin from the drumsticks and pull as much chicken as possible off the bone. Shred the chicken meat and return it to the pan. Remove from the heat and stir in the parsley.

Fresh Garden Soup

169 calories

Serves 4 • Ready in 1 hour

1 tsp olive oil (27 cals)
....
1 small onion, peeled and
chopped (36 cals)
....
2 garlic cloves, peeled and
finely sliced (6 cals)
....
1 leek, trimmed and cut into
fine rings (26 cals)
....
1 carrot, peeled and chopped
into large chunks (35 cals)
....
1 medium parsnip, peeled and
chopped into large chunks (51 cals)
....
2 celery sticks, trimmed
and chopped (10 cals)
....
1 sweet potato, peeled and chopped
into large chunks (124 cals)
....
1 × 400g (14oz) can chopped
tomatoes (64 cals)
....
1 bay leaf
....
1 handful of fresh parsley,
roughly chopped
....
1 chicken or vegetable stock cube (35 cals)
....
80g (3¼oz) frozen peas (53 cals)
....
1 x 400g (14oz) can cannellini beans,
drained and rinsed (210 cals)
....
salt and freshly ground black pepper
....

- Heat the olive oil in a medium-sized lidded saucepan, add the onion and garlic and fry very gently for 5 minutes. Add the leek, carrots, parsnip, celery and sweet potato and stir well.

- Add the canned tomatoes and bay leaf to the pan, then crumble in the stock cube. Top up with about 500ml (2 cups) water.

- Bring the mixture to the boil, cover with a lid, then reduce the heat and simmer very gently on the lowest heat for 45 minutes. Add the peas and cannellini beans and simmer for a further 5 minutes or until the peas are cooked. Season with salt and pepper to taste and serve.

Savoy Cabbage And Bacon Soup

222 calories

Serves 4 • Ready in 30 minutes

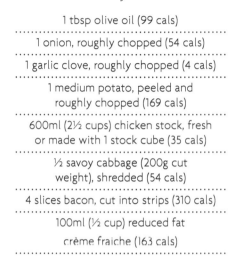

1 tbsp olive oil (99 cals)

1 onion, roughly chopped (54 cals)

1 garlic clove, roughly chopped (4 cals)

1 medium potato, peeled and
roughly chopped (169 cals)

600ml (2½ cups) chicken stock, fresh
or made with 1 stock cube (35 cals)

½ savoy cabbage (200g cut
weight), shredded (54 cals)

4 slices bacon, cut into strips (310 cals)

100ml (½ cup) reduced fat
crème fraiche (163 cals)

- Heat the oil in a large saucepan and gently fry the onions and garlic for 5 minutes. Add the potato and stock, bring to the boil and simmer for 10 minutes. Add the cabbage and cook for a further 5 minutes.

- Transfer to a blender (possibly in two batches) and blend until smooth. Re-heat the soup gently in the pan. In a separate frying pan dry fry the bacon strips until slightly brown on both sides (4- 5 minutes). Stir the bacon and crème fraiche into the soup.

Butternut Soup With Goat's Cheese

226 calories

Serves 2 • Ready in 45 minutes

1 tsp olive oil (27 cals)

1 garlic clove, peeled and crushed (4 cals)

450g (1lb) (cut weight) butternut
squash, cubed (190 cals)

2 spring onions (scallions), trimmed
and chopped (10 cals)

850ml (4 cups) vegetable stock (fresh
or made with 1 cube) (35 cals)

100g (3½oz) baby spinach (25 cals)

50g (¼ cup) soft goat's cheese,
chopped into cubes (160 cals)

freshly ground black pepper

- Heat the olive oil in a large saucepan and lightly fry the garlic. Add the butternut squash and spring onions (scallions) and stir through before adding the stock.

- Bring up to a simmer and cook for 30 minutes.

- Allow to cool slightly before transferring to a blender and blending until smooth.

- Reheat gently on the hob and stir in the spinach. Serve immediately with the goat's cheese on top and lashings of black pepper.

Chorizo And Tomato Soup

233 calories

Serves 4 • Ready in 45 minutes

1 tsp olive oil (27 cals)
....
1 onion, diced (54 cals)
....
1 garlic clove, finely sliced (4 cals)
....
1 green (bell) pepper, seeded
and diced (24 cals)
....
100g (3½oz) chorizo, diced (481 cals)
....
500ml (generous 2 cups)
vegetable stock, fresh or made
with one stock cube (35 cals)
....
1 x 400g (14oz) can chopped
tomatoes (64 cals)
....
300g (10½oz) passata (strained
tomatoes) (93 cals)
....
1 x 400g (14oz) can chick peas,
rinsed and drained (276 cals)
....

- Heat the oil in a saucepan, add the onion and cook gently for 5 minutes. Add the garlic, green pepper and chorizo, then cook for a further 5 minutes. Add the stock, tomatoes, passata and chick peas, then simmer for 30 minutes.

Lentil, Lemon And Thyme Soup

233 calories

Serves 4 • Ready in 45 minutes

1 tsp olive oil (27 cals)

1 large onion, finely diced (84 cals)

1 garlic clove, finely chopped (4 cals)

200g (1 cup) red lentils (678 cals)

1¼ litres (5 cups) vegetable stock,
fresh or made from 2 cubes (70 cals)

1 x 400g (14oz) can tomatoes,
chopped (64 cals)

2 tsp dried thyme, or 2 fresh sprigs

zest and juice of 1 lemon (4 cals)

- Heat the oil in a large saucepan and gently fry the onions and garlic for 5 minutes until soft. Add the lentils and stir into the onions. Pour in the stock, then bring to the boil. Simmer vigorously for 10 minutes.
- Reduce the heat and add the canned tomatoes, thyme and lemon zest. Bring back to a quiet simmer and cook gently for 30 minutes. Add the lemon juice and season to taste.

Hearty Ham Soup

256 calories

Serves 4 • Ready in 1 hour

1 tsp olive oil (27 cals)

1 large onion, peeled and diced (86 cals)

2 medium carrots, peeled
and diced (70 cals)

50g (1¾oz) pearl barley, rinsed (180 cals)

1 litre (4 cups) chicken stock, fresh or
made with 2 stock cubes (70 cals)

50g (1¾oz) Puy (French green)
lentils, rinsed (148 cals)

1 medium potato, peeled and
chopped into small dice (169 cals)

250g (9oz) cooked ham,
shredded (268 cals)

1 small handful of fresh parsley,
roughly chopped (3 cals)

- Heat the olive oil in a wide saucepan or casserole over a low heat. Add the onion and carrots and fry very gently for 10 minutes until the onion is translucent. Stir the pearl barley into the pan and pour in the stock. Bring to the boil, then reduce the heat and simmer for 30 minutes.

- Add the lentils and diced potato, top up with 1 litre (4 cups) water and cook for a further 30 minutes.

- Add the shredded ham to the pan and cook for a further 5 minutes. Stir in the parsley just before serving.

Spicy Ramen With Rice Noodles

258 calories

Serves 2 • Ready in 10 minutes

50g (2 heaped tablespoons)
Miso paste (101 cals)

....

2 tsp mirin (8 cals)

....

2 tbsp dark soy sauce (8 cals)

....

1 x 2.5cm (1 inch) fresh ginger,
peeled and grated (10 cals)

....

100g (4oz) spring greens or savoy
cabbage, shredded (28 cals)

....

1 carrot, peeled and cut into
very fine batons (35 cals)

....

100g (4oz) Shiitake mushrooms,
washed and sliced (24 cals)

....

100g (4oz) beansprouts (32 cals)

....

200g (7oz) fresh rice noodles (270 cals)

....

- Bring 750ml (3 cups) water to boiling point in a saucepan. Stir in the miso paste, mirin, soy and ginger. Stir until the miso is dissolved. Add in the greens, carrot and mushrooms. Put the lid on the pan and simmer gently for 5 minutes.

- Add the beansprouts and rice noodles to the ramen. Cook for a further 2 minutes before serving.

Minestrone

276 calories

Serves 4 • Ready in 30 minutes

1 tbsp olive oil (99 cals)

1 onion, chopped (54 cals)

2 carrots, peeled and chopped (70 cals)

3 celery sticks, trimmed
and chopped (15 cals)

2 garlic cloves, peeled and
finely chopped (8 cals)

2 tbsp tomato paste (60 cals)

1 x 400g (14oz) tin chopped
tomatoes (64 cals)

1¼ litres (5 cups) vegetable stock
(made from 2 cubes) (70 cals)

1 bay leaf

400g (14oz) tin cannellini beans,
drained and rinsed (259 cals)

100g (3½oz) conchiglie
(shell) pasta (354 cals)

75g (3oz) frozen peas (50 cals)

salt and pepper

- Heat the olive oil in a large saucepan over a low heat. Add the onion, carrot and celery and fry gently for 10 minutes. Stir in the garlic and tomato paste and fry for another 2 minutes.

- Add the tinned tomatoes, stock and bay leaf. Bring to a simmer and cook gently for 15 minutes.

- Add the cannellini beans, pasta and peas and cook for a further 10 minutes, or until the pasta is cooked. Remove the bay leaf and season with salt and pepper before serving.

Chicken and Fish

Tiger Prawns With Aïoli - 167 cals

Coriander And Lemon Chicken - 199 cals

Oriental Chicken With Mango - 234 cals

Hot And Sweet Chicken Curry - 235 cals

Chicken Satay - 244 cals

Baked Salmon With Asparagus - 271 cals

Seared Scallops With Garlicky Potatoes - 308 cals

Wasabi Salmon - 310 cals

Fragrant Chicken - 333 cals

Crunchy Tuna Bake - 342 cals

Lightly Spiced Prawns & Vegetable Rice - 357 cals

Crispy Baked Chicken - 366 cals

One Pot Lemon Chicken - 395 cals

Chicken, Rice And Peas - 399 cals

Spicy Chicken Flatbread - 399 cals

Chinese Chicken Stir-Fry - 429 cals

Egg Fried Rice With Prawns - 432 cals

Tomato Chicken Spaghetti - 434 cals

Light Chicken Stew - 435 cals

Chicken & Broccoli in White Wine - 445 cals

Thai Chicken Curry - 449 cals

Spicy Prawn Stir-Fry - 456 cals

Turkey Meatballs in Tomato Sauce - 452 cals

Peanut Butter And Lime Prawns - 441 cals

Chicken Tikka Masala - 456 cals

Steamed Salmon With Spicy Rice - 468 cals

Tiger Prawns With Aïoli

167 calories

Serves 2 • Ready in 20 minutes

225g (8oz) raw tiger prawns (jumbo
shrimp) (171 cals) juice of ½ lemon (2 cals)

For the marinade:

2 garlic cloves, peeled and finely
chopped (6 cals) grated zest of 1 lemon

1 tbsp olive oil (99 cals)

1 tsp finely chopped fresh parsley salt
and freshly ground black pepper

For the aïoli:

Juice of ½ lemon (2 cals)

½ tsp saffron threads

½ garlic clove, peeled and
finely chopped (2 cals)

3 tbsp (50ml) white wine (33 cals)

2 tbsp extra-light mayonnaise (30 cals)

- To make the marinade, mix the garlic, lemon zest, olive oil, parsley and salt and pepper to taste together in a large bowl.

- Add the prawns (shrimp) and coat well with the marinade. Leave to marinate in the refrigerator for at least 15 minutes.

- To make the aïoli, place the lemon juice, saffron, garlic and white wine in a saucepan. Bring to the boil, then reduce the heat and simmer for a few minutes. Place the mayonnaise in a bowl, pour in the lemon juice mixture and stir well.

- When you are ready to cook the prawns, light the barbecue or preheat the grill (broiler) to high, then grill (broil) the prawns for 1–2 minutes on each side until cooked through. Pile the prawns in a bowl and squeeze the lemon juice over the top. Serve with the aïoli on the side.

Coriander And Lemon Chicken

199 calories

Serves 1 • Ready in 45 minutes

1 × 150g (5oz) skinless, boneless
chicken breast, cut in half and scored
lightly with a knife (159 cals)

Zest and juice of ½ lemon (8 cals)

½ garlic clove, peeled and crushed (2 cals)

1 handful of fresh coriander (cilantro)
leaves, chopped (4 cals)

1 tsp olive oil (27 cals)

salt and freshly ground black pepper

- Wash the lemon in hot soapy water (only if waxed) and dry on kitchen paper (paper towels). Using the fine side of the grater, grate a little of the zest of the lemon into a medium-sized bowl. Add the garlic, coriander (cilantro) leaves, olive oil and the juice of the ½ lemon. Mix together with a little salt and pepper.

- Put the chicken into the marinade and use your fingers to rub the marinade all over until the chicken is coated. Cover and leave to rest in the refrigerator for at least 15 minutes.

- Heat a griddle pan or frying pan (skillet) over a medium-high heat. Add the chicken, press it into the pan and cook for about 6–8 minutes on each side, turning the heat down if it looks like it's starting to catch, until the chicken is cooked through. Leave to rest in the pan for 2 minutes before serving.

Oriental Chicken With Mango

234 calories

Serves 2 • Ready in 20 minutes

2 × 150g (5oz) skinless, boneless chicken
breasts, cut in half lengthways (318 cals)
....
½ tsp chopped fresh rosemary
....
½ tsp chopped fresh thyme
....
salt and freshly ground black pepper
....
1 tsp olive oil (27 cals)
....
100g (3½oz) mango pieces, chopped
into small pieces (65 cals)
....
2 tsp brown sugar (36 cals)
....
1 tbsp red wine vinegar (2 cals)
....
1 tbsp dry sherry (14 cals)
....
1 small thumb fresh root ginger,
peeled and finely grated (5 cals)
....

- Rub the chicken breast pieces with the herbs and a little salt and pepper.

- Heat the olive oil in a large frying pan (skillet) over a medium heat. Add the chicken and fry until golden brown and cooked through, about 8–10 minutes on each side. Remove the chicken from the pan with a slotted spoon, cover and keep warm.

- Return the pan to a medium heat, add the mango and fry for 2 minutes, then add the sugar, vinegar, sherry and ginger, stir well and continue to fry for a further 2 minutes. Pour the mango sauce over the chicken to serve.

Hot And Sweet Chicken Curry

235 calories

Serves 2 • Ready in 30 minutes

2 tsp sunflower oil (54 cals)

....

1 medium onion, peeled and
finely chopped (65 cals)

....

2 bird's eye (Thai) chillies,
finely chopped (1 cal)

....

3 garlic cloves, peeled and grated (9 cals)

....

2.5cm (1in) piece fresh root ginger,
peeled and grated (5 cals)

....

a pinch of salt

....

1 tomato, diced (14 cals)

....

2 × 150g (5oz) skinless, boneless chicken
breasts, cut into cubes (318 cals)

....

½ tsp ground cumin

....

1 tsp coarsely ground black pepper

....

1 small handful of fresh coriander
(cilantro), chopped (3 cals)

....

- Heat the oil in a wide frying pan (skillet) over a medium-high heat. When hot, add the onion, chillies, garlic, ginger and salt and stir-fry for 2 minutes before reducing the heat and cooking gently for a further 5 minutes.

- Increase the heat to medium, toss in the tomato and stir-fry for 2 minutes. Add the chicken, cumin and pepper and stir-fry for a further 5 minutes.

- Reduce the heat to low, pour in 150ml (^{2}/^{3} cup) water, stir and cook for another 5 minutes. If there seems to be too much liquid, increase the heat and boil for 1–2 minutes. Stir in the coriander (cilantro) before serving.

Chicken Satay

244 calories

Serves 2 • Ready in 15 minutes, plus 3–4 hours marinating

1 shallot, peeled and diced (5 cals)
1 garlic clove, peeled and crushed (3 cals)
2 tsp curry powder
1 level tbsp peanut butter (182 cals)
1 tsp runny honey (23 cals)
2 tbsp soy sauce (9 cals)
250g (9oz) skinless, boneless chicken breast, cut into cubes, about 2.5cm (1in) square (265 cals)

- To make the marinade, mix the shallot, garlic, curry powder, peanut butter, honey and soy sauce together in a bowl. Add the chicken and toss until the chicken is coated all over in the marinade. Leave to marinate in the refrigerator for 3–4 hours.

- Preheat the grill (broiler) to medium or light the barbecue. Thread the chicken cubes onto 2–4 skewers, leaving room between the chicken pieces to allow them to cook thoroughly. Grill (broil) for about 10 minutes, turning regularly, until cooked through. Serve immediately.

Baked Salmon With Asparagus

271 calories

Serves 1 • Ready in 20 minutes

1 × 120g (4oz) skinless salmon fillet (216 cals)
1 fresh rosemary sprig
1 fresh sage leaf
4 black peppercorns
1 star anise
½ lemongrass stalk
1 garlic clove, unpeeled and cut in half (3 cals)
2 thick slices lemon
1 tsp olive oil (27 cals)
100g (3½oz) fine asparagus (25 cals)
lemon juice, for drizzling

- Preheat the oven to 190C/fan 170C/375F.

- Place a piece of foil on a baking tray and place the salmon in the middle of the foil. Put the rosemary, sage, peppercorns, star anise, lemongrass and garlic around the fish. Put the lemon slices on top and drizzle with the olive oil. Fold the foil around the salmon to make a shallow tent.

- Cook the salmon in the oven for 8 minutes, then add the asparagus and return to the oven for a further 8 minutes. Remove from the oven and leave to rest for 2 minutes before serving.

- Arrange the asparagus on a warmed serving plate and place the salmon on top. Drizzle a little lemon juice over the dish and serve.

Seared Scallops With Garlicky Potatoes

308 calories

Serves 2 • Ready in 20 minutes

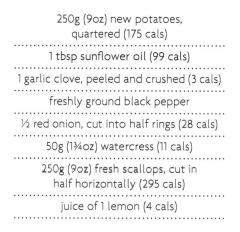

250g (9oz) new potatoes,
quartered (175 cals)
....
1 tbsp sunflower oil (99 cals)
....
1 garlic clove, peeled and crushed (3 cals)
....
freshly ground black pepper
....
½ red onion, cut into half rings (28 cals)
....
50g (1¾oz) watercress (11 cals)
....
250g (9oz) fresh scallops, cut in
half horizontally (295 cals)
....
juice of 1 lemon (4 cals)
....

- Boil the potatoes for 12-15 minutes until just cooked through. Drain then leave to cool slightly on kitchen paper (paper towels) and blot dry.

- Heat the oil in a frying pan (skillet) over a medium heat and fry the potatoes, garlic and black pepper together until the potatoes are just browning. Remove the potato and garlicky goodness from the pan and place in a bowl with the red onion and watercress.

- Wipe the pan with kitchen paper to remove any excess oil and heat the pan over a high heat. When hot, add the scallops and fry for 1–2 minutes. They should be seared on both sides and just cooked through.

- Toss the cooked scallops into the potatoes and squeeze on the lemon juice before serving.

Wasabi Salmon

310 calories

Serves 1 • Ready in 20 minutes

1 skinless salmon fillet, about
130g (4½oz) (234 cals)

....

1 tsp wasabi paste (13 cals)

....

1 tbsp natural yogurt (22 cals)

....

1 tbsp rice wine vinegar (3 cals)

....

2 fresh mint leaves, finely chopped

....

salt and freshly ground black pepper

....

1 × 80g (3oz) bag baby leaf
or herb salad (16 cals)

....

2 radishes, thinly sliced (2 cals)

....

5cm (2in) piece cucumber, halved
lengthways and sliced (10 cals)

....

2 spring onions (scallions),
trimmed and sliced (10 cals)

....

- Preheat the oven to 200C/180C fan/400F.

- Place the salmon fillet on a baking tray and bake in the oven for 16–18 minutes until just cooked through. Remove from the oven and set aside. When it has cooled for just a few minutes, rub the wasabi paste over the top.

- In a small bowl, mix the yogurt, vinegar, mint and salt and pepper together and leave to stand for at least 5 minutes to allow the flavours to develop.

- Arrange the salad leaves on a serving plate and top with the radishes, cucumber and spring onions (scallions). Flake the salmon over the top and drizzle the dressing over.

Fragrant Chicken

333 calories

Serves 2 • Ready in 30 minutes

1 tsp olive oil (27 cals)
....
1 small onion, chopped (22 cals)
....
½ tsp cumin seeds
....
½ tsp turmeric
....
300ml (1¼ cups) fresh
chicken stock (21 cals)
....
½ lemon (2 cals)
....
2 × 150g (5oz) skinless chicken
breasts, diced (318 cals)
....
200g (7oz) new potatoes, quartered (140 cals)
....
few strands of saffron
....
10g (2 tsp) butter (74 cals)
....
12 large black olives, pitted (62 cals)
....
4 fresh basil leaves, roughly chopped
....
salt and freshly ground black pepper
....

- Heat the oil in a pan over a low heat, add the onion and sweat for 7–8 minutes. Add the cumin seeds and turmeric and fry for 1–2 minutes until aromatic.

- Pour in the chicken stock and bring to a gentle simmer. Add the lemon zest then cut out the flesh of the lemon, roughly chop and add to the pan. Add the chicken, potatoes and saffron. Bring back to simmering point and cook gently for 10 minutes until the potatoes are tender and the chicken is cooked through. Remove the chicken and potatoes from the pan and keep warm.

- Increase the heat under the pan to high and stir in the butter, olives, basil and salt and pepper. Bubble over a high heat for 2–4 minutes until the sauce is a little thicker and glossy. Pour the sauce over the chicken and potatoes and serve immediately.

Crunchy Tuna Bake

342 calories

Serves 2 • Ready in one hour

300g (11oz) new potatoes (about 7
medium), with skin on (210 cals)

1 × 200g (7oz) can tuna steaks
in water, drained (148 cals)

1 courgette (zucchini), peeled
and finely diced (27 cals)

40 ripe cherry tomatoes, halved (90 cals)

1 garlic clove, peeled and chopped (3 cals)

2 tbsp tomato purée (paste) mixed
with 2 tbsp water (61 cals)

1 tsp olive oil (27 cals)

20g panko breadcrumbs (75 cals)

10g (1/3oz) Parmesan cheese,
finely grated (42 cals)

freshly ground black pepper

- Boil or steam the new potatoes for 20 minutes until tender, then drain and leave until cool enough to handle.

- Preheat the oven to 190C/fan 170C/375F.

- In a small ovenproof baking dish, arrange the tuna, courgette (zucchini) and tomatoes across the bottom, making sure the majority of the tomatoes are cut side up. Sprinkle the chopped garlic over the top, then pour in the tomato paste mixture.

- When the potatoes are cool, slice them as thinly as possible; the slices should be 2–3mm (1/8in) thick. Arrange the potatoes on top of the tuna mixture, allowing them to overlap, then brush the top with the olive oil and sprinkle over the breadcrumbs, Parmesan and pepper to taste.

- Cook in the oven for 30 minutes, then serve.

Lightly Spiced Prawns With Vegetable Rice

357 calories

Serves 2 • Ready in 20 minutes

80g (3oz) basmati rice (282 cals)

1 tsp olive oil

1 clove

1 bay leaf

1 small onion, peeled and chopped (35 cals)

1 green (bell) pepper, deseeded and chopped (24 cals)

2 cloves garlic, peeled and thinly sliced (8 cals)

1 red or green chilli, deseeded and sliced (optional)

½ tsp mild chilli powder

½ tsp paprika (7 cals)

¼ tsp ground turmeric

¼ tsp ground cumin

¼ tsp cinnamon

1 tsp salt

2 fresh tomatoes, roughly chopped (28 cals)

60g (2oz) frozen edamame beans (82 cals)

1 tbsp water

225g (8oz) raw king prawns (if frozen, cook for a little longer/defrost as per pack instructions) (234 cals)

60g (2oz) young leaf spinach,

stalks removed (14 cals)
....
Small handful fresh coriander
(cilantro), chopped
....

- Cook the rice by your preferred method.

- In a wide lidded frying pan, heat the oil on a medium heat. Add the cloves and bay leaf. Add the onion and red pepper. Stir, turn the heat to low and place the lid on the pan. Cook for 5 minutes.

- Remove the lid from the pan. Add the garlic, chilli, chilli powder, paprika, turmeric, ground cumin, cinnamon and salt and fry for a further minute. Add the chopped tomatoes, edamame beans and water. Replace the lid on the pan and cook gently for 7 minutes.

- Take the lid off the pan and remove the cloves and bay leaf. Add the prawns and cook until just pink. Then add the rice, stir thoroughly and warm through. Finally, stir through the spinach and coriander just before serving.

Crispy Baked Chicken

366 calories

Serves 2 • Ready in 20 minutes

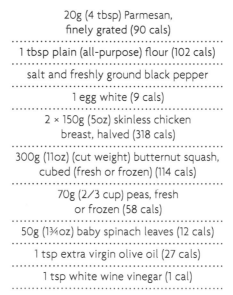

20g (4 tbsp) Parmesan,
finely grated (90 cals)

....

1 tbsp plain (all-purpose) flour (102 cals)

....

salt and freshly ground black pepper

....

1 egg white (9 cals)

....

2 × 150g (5oz) skinless chicken
breast, halved (318 cals)

....

300g (11oz) (cut weight) butternut squash,
cubed (fresh or frozen) (114 cals)

....

70g (2/3 cup) peas, fresh
or frozen (58 cals)

....

50g (1¾oz) baby spinach leaves (12 cals)

....

1 tsp extra virgin olive oil (27 cals)

....

1 tsp white wine vinegar (1 cal)

....

- Preheat the oven to 200C/180C Fan/400F

- Loosely mix the Parmesan, flour and a little salt and pepper on a plate. Beat the egg white in a wide bowl.

- Dip each piece of chicken first in the egg white and then in the Parmesan, making sure it is lightly coated on both sides.

- Place the chicken pieces on a baking tray and arrange the butternut squash around them. Bake for 15-20 minutes or until the chicken is cooked through.

- Cook the peas in boiling water for 6 minutes until tender.

- Drain the peas and return to the pan. Stir through the spinach, allowing it to wilt slightly in the heat. Add the olive oil and vinegar and stir through.

- Transfer to 2 serving plates and arrange the chicken and butternut squash on top of the green vegetables.

One Pot Lemon Chicken

395 calories

Serves 4 • Ready in 30 minutes

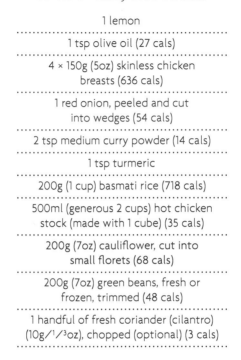

1 lemon
....
1 tsp olive oil (27 cals)
....
4 × 150g (5oz) skinless chicken
breasts (636 cals)
....
1 red onion, peeled and cut
into wedges (54 cals)
....
2 tsp medium curry powder (14 cals)
....
1 tsp turmeric
....
200g (1 cup) basmati rice (718 cals)
....
500ml (generous 2 cups) hot chicken
stock (made with 1 cube) (35 cals)
....
200g (7oz) cauliflower, cut into
small florets (68 cals)
....
200g (7oz) green beans, fresh or
frozen, trimmed (48 cals)
....
1 handful of fresh coriander (cilantro)
(10g/¹/³oz), chopped (optional) (3 cals)
....

- Wash the lemon in hot soapy water and dry. Cut in half lengthways and then cut into very thin slices.

- Using a large lidded frying pan (skillet) or casserole dish, heat the oil over a medium–high heat. When hot, add the chicken and red onion and brown the chicken on all sides. Stir in the curry powder, turmeric and rice, then pour in the hot stock.

- Add the cauliflower, beans and sliced lemon to the pan. Bring to the boil, reduce the heat and simmer with the lid on for 10 minutes. The chicken should be cooked through and the rice tender. Stir in the coriander (cilantro) and serve.

Chicken, Rice And Peas

399 calories

Serves 1 • Ready in 15 minutes

30g (scant ¼ cup) basmati rice
(dry weight) (108 cals)
....
50g (scant ½ cup) frozen peas (33 cals)
....
few sprays of light oil spray (3 cals)
....
1 × 150g (5oz) skinless chicken
breast, cut into strips (159 cals)
....
75ml (1/3 cup) skimmed
(skim) milk (28 cals)
....
½ tbsp light soft cheese (27 cals)
....
10g (2 tbsp) mature (sharp)
Cheddar, grated (41 cals)
....
salt and freshly ground black pepper
....

- Boil the rice as per the packet instructions. Add the frozen peas 6 minutes before the end of the cooking time. Drain and set aside.

- Heat the spray oil in a frying pan (skillet) over a medium heat and fry the chicken for 8-10 minutes, until browned all over and just cooked through.

- Add the milk, soft cheese and Cheddar to the frying pan. Bring to a gentle simmer and continue to cook gently for 5 minutes.

- Finally, add the cooked rice and peas to the pan and heat through. Season with salt and pepper.

- Serve immediately.

Spicy Chicken Flatbread

399 calories

Serves 1 • Ready in 15 minutes

1 × 150g (5oz) skinless chicken breast,
cut into 4–5 slices (159 cals)

....

½ level tbsp plain (all-purpose)
flour (34 cals)

....

salt and freshly ground black pepper

....

½ tsp paprika (3 cals)

....

1 tsp olive oil (27 cals)

....

100g (3½oz) bag baby leaf salad (21 cals)

....

100g (3½oz) cucumber
(about 5cm/2in piece),

....

roughly chopped (10 cals)

....

10 cherry tomatoes, halved (22 cals)

....

1 tbsp natural plain yogurt (22 cals)

....

¼ tsp paprika (2 cals)

....

1 flatbread (99 cals)

....

- Place the chicken in a bowl and sprinkle on the flour, salt and pepper and ½ teaspoon paprika. Use your hands to toss the chicken in the flour and make sure it is evenly covered.

- Heat the oil in a frying pan (skillet) over a medium heat. When hot, add the chicken and fry for about 4 minutes on each side, depending on thickness.

- Cook your flatbread under the grill (or follow the instructions on the packet).

- Meanwhile, prepare all your salad ingredients. Combine the yogurt and ¼ teaspoon paprika in a small cup.

- Layer up the flatbread with the salad first, then the chicken and finally the yogurt dressing drizzled over.

Chinese Chicken Stir-Fry

429 calories

Serves 2 • Ready in 20 minutes

1 small egg white (7 cals)

2 tsp cornflour (cornstarch) (36 cals)

2 × 150g (5oz) skinless chicken
breasts, cut into strips (318 cals)

1 tsp Thai fish sauce (nam pla) (4 cals)

juice of 1 lime (4 cals)

1 tsp vegetable oil (27 cals)

½ red (bell) pepper, deseeded and cut into
large chunks (27 cals)

2.5cm (1in) piece of fresh ginger,
peeled and grated (20 cals)

1 shallot, peeled and thinly sliced (6 cals)

1 garlic clove, peeled and
thinly sliced (3 cals)

1 red chilli, deseeded and sliced (2 cals)

300g (11oz) bag mixed vegetable
stir-fry (158 cals)

150g (5oz) quick cook egg
noodles (246 cals)

8 fresh basil leaves

- Whisk together the egg white and 1 teaspoon of cornflour (cornstarch) with a fork. Tip in the chicken and stir to coat. Leave to marinate for 5 minutes.

- Remove the chicken from the marinade and pat dry with kitchen paper (paper towels).

- Combine the fish sauce, lime juice, 2 tablespoons water and the rest of the cornflour.

- Heat the oil in a wok or wide heavy-based frying pan (skillet) over a medium–high heat. When hot, toss in the chicken and stir-fry for 8-10 minutes until just cooked. Remove the chicken from the pan.

- Turn the heat to maximum and stir-fry the (bell) pepper, ginger, shallot, garlic and chilli. Add the bagged veg and stir-fry for 4 minutes.

- Turn the heat down a little and add the egg noodles. Stir for 2 minutes.

- Pour in the fish sauce mix and add the chicken and basil leaves. Heat through and serve immediately.

- Add the cauliflower, beans and sliced lemon to the pan. Bring to the boil, reduce the heat and simmer with the lid on for 10 minutes. The chicken should be cooked through and the rice tender. Stir in the coriander (cilantro) and serve.

Egg Fried Rice With Prawns

432 calories

Serves 2 • Ready in 15 minutes

80g (3oz) basmati rice (282 cals)

40g (1½oz) frozen peas (27 cals)

2 tsp olive oil (54 cals)

3 large free-range eggs, beaten (297 cals)

3 spring onions (scallions), trimmed
and shredded (14 cals)

½ garlic clove, peeled and
finely chopped (2 cals)

225g (8oz) cooked prawns
(shrimp) (171 cals)

1 tbsp dry sherry (14 cals)

1 small handful of fresh coriander
(cilantro) leaves, chopped (3 cals)

salt and freshly ground black pepper

- Cook the rice by your preferred method and add the peas for the last 5 minutes of cooking time.

- Heat 1 teaspoon of olive oil in a wide saucepan or wok, add the eggs and scramble lightly, removing them from the pan while they are still a little runny and just before they are fully cooked. Transfer to a bowl, cover and set aside.

- Heat the remaining oil, add the spring onions (scallions) and garlic and gently fry for a minute, then add the prawns (shrimp) and fry for a further minute. Add the sherry and coriander (cilantro), season with salt and pepper and then add the rice and peas. Cook for a further minute before stirring through the lightly scrambled eggs and serve immediately.

Tomato Chicken Spaghetti

434 calories

Serves 2 • Ready in 20 minutes

2 × 150g (5oz) skinless, boneless chicken breasts (318 cals)
1 tbsp tomato purée (paste) (30 cals)
1 tsp chopped fresh basil
1 tsp olive oil (27 cals)
1 garlic clove, peeled and finely sliced (3 cals)
1 × 400g (14oz) can whole tomatoes (64 cals)
a pinch of salt
1 tbsp red wine vinegar (1 cal)
120g (4oz) wholewheat spaghetti (424 calories)

- Cut each chicken breast into 2 pieces and lightly score on both sides. Rub the tomato purée (paste) and half the basil over the 4 pieces of chicken and leave to rest while you prepare the sauce.

- Heat the olive oil gently in a non-stick saucepan, add the garlic and fry for 1–2 minutes until just starting to brown. Add the canned tomatoes, salt and the remaining basil and simmer over a medium heat for 10 minutes. Reduce the heat and break up the tomatoes with the back of a wooden spoon. Add the red wine vinegar and continue to simmer gently for another 10 min.

- Meanwhile, preheat the grill (broiler) to medium. Arrange the chicken pieces on the grill pan and grill (broil) for 7–8 minutes on each side. The chicken should be cooked through and golden.

- Cook the spaghetti as per the pack instructions and divide between 2 bowls.

- Add the chicken to the tomato sauce and stir in. Heat for a further 2–3 minutes, then serve over the spaghetti.

Light Chicken Stew

435 calories

Serves 2 • Ready in 1 hour

50g (¼ cup) chopped streaky
bacon or lardons (138 cals)
....

2 skinless, boneless chicken thighs,
about 360g (12oz) (392 cals)
....

½ leek, trimmed and roughly
chopped (13 cals)
....

1 celery stick, finely sliced (2 cals)
....

2 garlic cloves, peeled and
finely sliced (6 cals)
....

1 tsp mixed dried herbs (8 cals)
....

200ml (generous ¾ cup) good
quality cider (72 cals)
....

80g (¾ cup) frozen peas (53 cals)
....

200g (7oz) new potatoes (about 4 med),
with skin on, quartered (140 cals)
....

1 tbsp Dijon mustard (28 cals)
....

salt and freshly ground black pepper
....

1 Little Gem (Boston) lettuce,
roughly shredded (17 cals)
....

- Heat the chopped bacon or lardons in a heavy based lidded saucepan, cooking them until they brown all over. Remove them from the pan with a slotted spoon and set aside. Add the chicken thighs and cook on the first side for about 5 minutes over a medium heat.

- Turn the chicken over and add the leek, celery, garlic and dried herbs. Give everything a stir and let it continue to cook for a further 5 minutes. Return the chopped bacon or lardons to the pan.

- Pour in the cider and add the peas and potatoes. Bring to the boil, then reduce the heat, put the lid on and cook for 20–30 minutes until the chicken is cooked through.
- Remove the lid, stir in the mustard and season with salt and pepper. Finally, toss the lettuce over the chicken and let it wilt into the sauce for about 2 minutes.

Chicken and Tenderstem Broccoli in White Wine

445 calories

Serves 2 • Ready in 15 minutes

80g (3oz) basmati rice (282 cals)
1 tsp olive oil (27 cals)
1 garlic clove, peeled and crushed (4 cals)
2 spring onions (scallions), trimmed and sliced (10 cals)
½ tsp dried mixed herbs
2 × 150g (5oz) skinless chicken breast, both halved (318 cals)
150g tenderstem broccoli, trimmed (62 cals)
200ml (1 cup) dry white wine (132 cals)
2 tbsp light soft cheese (50 cals)
handful of fresh parsley, chopped (4 cals)

- Cook the rice by your preferred method. Divide between 2 bowls.

- Heat the oil, garlic, spring onions (scallions) and dried mixed herbs in a small lidded frying pan (skillet) or saucepan for 1–2 minutes until sizzling. Add the chicken and cook for about 4 minutes until the first side turns golden.

- Turn the chicken over and add the broccoli and white wine. Put the lid on and as soon as it starts to simmer, turn the heat to low. Let the chicken continue to cook in the wine for a further 5 minutes. Check that the chicken is cooked through before removing the chicken and broccoli from the pan and covering.

- Bring the remaining liquid in the pan back up to simmering and stir in the soft cheese. Bubble for 2–3 minutes until you get a pleasingly thick sauce. Stir in the parsley.

- Arrange the chicken and broccoli over the rice & add the sauce.

Thai Chicken Curry

449 calories

Serves 2 • Ready in 15 minutes

80g (3oz) basmati rice (282 cals)

1 tsp sunflower oil (27 cals)

250g (9oz) skinless, boneless chicken
breast, cut into cubes, about
2.5cm (1in) square (265 cals)

1 tbsp Thai green curry paste (30 cals)

½ × 400ml (14oz) can light
coconut milk, stirred (146 cals)

1 red (bell) pepper, deseeded
and cut into strips (51 cals)

75g (3oz) frozen peas (50 cals)

2 spring onions (scallions), trimmed
and shredded (10 cals)

1 x 160g (5½oz) pak choi,
roughly chopped (30 cals)

juice of 1 lime (4 cals)

1 fresh basil leaf, shredded

1 small handful of fresh coriander
(cilantro) leaves, roughly chopped (3 cals)

- Cook the rice by your preferred method. Divide between 2 bowls.

- Warm the oil in a wide saucepan, and fry the chicken lightly.

- Add the curry paste and stir-fry for 1 minute before adding the coconut milk. Simmer for 2 minutes, then add the (bell) pepper, peas and spring onion (scallion) and simmer for a further 5 minutes, or until the peas are tender. Add the pak choi and and cook for 2 more minutes.

- Finally, stir in the lime juice, basil and coriander (cilantro) and serve over the rice.

Spicy Prawn Stir-Fry

456 calories

Serves 2 • Ready in 15 minutes

1 garlic clove, peeled and crushed (4 cals)

1 tsp tamarind paste (12 cals)

2 tbsp dark soy sauce (8 cals)

300g (10oz) cooked king prawns
(king shrimp) (296 cals)

1 tsp walnut oil (44 cals)

1 yellow (bell) pepper, deseeded
and cut into thin strips (42 cals)

1 red (bell) pepper, deseeded and
cut into thin strips (54 cals)

1 red chilli, deseeded and cut
into fine rings (3 cals)

100g (3oz) beansprouts (32 cals)

100g (3oz) mangetout (snow peas) (32 cals)

300g (11oz) fresh rice noodles (384 cals)

- Mix the garlic, tamarind paste and soy sauce together in a bowl. Add the prawns (shrimp) and turn until they are coated all over in the dark sticky mixture. Leave to stand for 2 minutes while you prepare the rest of the stir-fry.

- Heat the walnut oil in a wok or large frying pan (skillet) over a high heat, add the (bell) peppers and chilli and stir-fry for 3 minutes. Add the beansprouts and mangetout (snow peas) and stir-fry for a further 2 minutes.

- Reduce the heat to medium and add the prawns and marinade and stir-fry for a further 2 minutes until the prawns are warmed through. Then stir in the rice noodles for 2 minutes before serving.

Sweet Italian Turkey Meatballs in Tomato Sauce

452 calories

Serves 4 • Ready in 20 minutes + 10 mins chill time

500g (1lb 2oz) turkey thigh mince (ground turkey thigh) (755 cals)
1 tsp salt
1 tsp pepper
1 tsp oregano
1 tsp Dried mixed herbs
1 tsp paprika (14 cals)
1 tsp mild chilli powder
2 cloves garlic, crushed (8 cals)
1 tbsp ketchup (29 cals)
500g (1lb 2oz) passata (strained tomatoes) (154 cals)
240g (8oz) wholewheat spaghetti (848 calories)

- Place the turkey in a mixing bowl. Add the salt, pepper, herbs, paprika, chilli powder, garlic, and ketchup.

- Use your hands to pound and mix the ingredients together. Use your fists to make sure the turkey is thoroughly broken up.

- Form the meat into 12 meatballs. Place on a tray in the freezer for 10 minutes or in the fridge for 30 minutes before cooking.

- To cook, lightly fry in a tbsp olive oil. Fry the meatballs for about 4 mins and then add the passata and bubble in sauce for about 10 minutes.

- Cook the spaghetti as per the pack instructions and spoon the sauce over.

Peanut Butter And Lime Prawns

441 calories

Serves 1 • Ready in 20 minutes

For the marinade:
....
Juice of ½ lime (2 cals)
....
1 tsp (10g) peanut butter (60 cals)
....
1 tbsp water
....
½ tsp tomato puree (paste) (4 cals)
....
½ clove garlic, crushed (2 cals)
....
¼ tsp ground ginger
....
125g (4oz) raw king prawns (130 cals)
....
For the rice:
....
30g (scant ¼ cup) basmati rice
(dry weight) (108 cals)
....
2 tomatoes, chopped (28 cals)
....
5cm (2 inches) cucumber, cut
into small cubes (10 cals)
....
1 spring onion (scallion),
finely chopped (5 cals)
....
Juice of ½ lime (2 cals)
....
Salt and pepper
....

- Firstly, cook the rice by your preferred method and leave to cool.

- Combine all the marinade ingredients in a wide bowl and stir together thoroughly. Add the king prawns and leave to marinate for 15-20 minutes.

- Place the cooked rice in a bowl and mush gently with a fork to remove any lumps. Add the tomatoes, cucumber and spring onion. Squeeze over the lime juice and season with salt and pepper. Stir well and leave for the flavours to develop.

- Remove the prawns from the marinade and shake off into the bowl so you don't lose any precious marinade. Place on kitchen paper to dry. Heat a frying pan on a medium heat and add the marinade. Heat gently and allow to bubble for 2 minutes, adding a little more water if necessary, before transferring to a small bowl for dipping.

- Turn the heat up to high and add the prawns. Fry for 3-4 minutes, stirring regularly until cooked through. To serve, place the rice on a plate and arrange the prawns over the top. Serve with the dipping sauce on the side.

Chicken Tikka Masala

456 calories

Serves 4 • Ready in 2 hours 30 minutes

1 medium onion, peeled (54 cals)

2 garlic cloves, peeled (6 cals)

2cm (1in) piece of fresh
ginger, peeled (10 cals)

1 tsp chilli (red pepper) flakes
(or hot chilli powder)

2 heaped tsp paprika (28 cals)

½ tsp ground coriander

½ tsp ground cumin

½ tsp ground turmeric

1 tsp salt

1 tbsp (20g) ground almonds (122 cals)

2 tbsp tomato purée (paste) (60 cals)

juice of 1 lime (4 cals)

2 tsp sunflower oil (54 cals)

200ml (generous ¾ cup) low-fat
plain yogurt (112 cals)

500g (1lb 2oz) skinless chicken breast,
cut into rough cubes (530 cals)

2 tbsp double (heavy) cream (269 cals)

160g (¾ cup) basmati rice (574 cals)

- Preheat the oven to 140C/120C fan/275F.

- Process the onion, garlic and ginger to a paste in a food processor or use a hand blender or grate using the large side of the grater for the onion and the fine side for the garlic and ginger. Either way they should be combined into a thick gloopy paste.

- Stir in the spices, salt and ground almonds, then add the tomato purée (paste) and lime juice and mix well.

- Heat the oil in a frying pan (skillet) over a medium heat for 2 minutes before adding in the paste. It should sizzle nicely. Stir-fry for 1 minute until it starts to release its spicy aroma. Turn the heat down and stir in the yogurt and bubble gently for 1–2 minutes.

- Place the diced chicken in the base of a casserole dish or your slow cooker and pour the sauce over.

- Cook in the oven for 2 hours or in your slow cooker on low for 5–6 hours. Stir in the cream at the end of the cooking time.

Steamed Salmon With Spicy Rice

468 calories

Serves 2 • Ready in 20 minutes

For the salmon:

½ tsp cumin seeds

few black peppercorns

bay leaf

2 skinless salmon fillets, about
130g (4½oz) each (468 cals)

For the rice:

1 tsp sunflower oil (27 cals)

½ tsp cumin seeds

½ tsp mustard seeds

1 tsp desiccated (dry unsweetened)
coconut (18 cals)

½ tsp chilli powder

¼ tsp ground ginger (3 cals)

½ tsp turmeric

½ tsp ground coriander

pinch of salt

80g (3oz) basmati rice (282 cals)

200ml (scant 1 cup) water

200g (7oz) kale, shredded (66 cals)

100g (scant 1 cup) frozen peas (66 cals)

generous handful of fresh
coriander (cilantro) (15g/½oz),
roughly chopped (4 cals)

juice of ½ lemon (2 cals)

- In a small saucepan, heat the cumin seeds until they start to sizzle and toast. Remove from the heat. Add the peppercorns and bay leaf to the pan then lay the salmon on the top. Add just enough water to the pan to cover the salmon and bring the water to the boil. When boiling, reduce the heat and cook for 5–6 minutes until the salmon is cooked through. Remove the salmon from the pan and set aside.

- For the rice, heat the oil in a large lidded frying pan (skillet) over a medium–high heat. Add the cumin seeds, mustard seeds and coconut and fry for 1 minute until sizzling nicely. Stir in the rest of the spices and then the rice and water.

- Bring up to a simmer, place the lid on the pan and cook for 8 minutes, or until the rice is nearly cooked.

- Add the kale and peas along with a little water if needed. Put the lid on the pan and cook slowly for 6 minutes until the kale and peas are just cooked. If necessary cook for a couple of minutes with the lid off to remove excess water. Flake the salmon into large chunks into the pan. Add the fresh coriander (cilantro) and lemon juice, then warm through for 1–2 minutes before serving.

Pork, Beef and Lamb

Zesty Pork Steaks With Mushrooms - 224 cals

Quick Italian Beef Stew - 229 cals

Asian-Style Stir-Fried Beef & Mushrooms - 267 cals

Minted Lamb with Butternut Crush - 303 cals

Lamb Tagine - 303 cals

Grilled Lamb & Tangy Lemon Couscous - 314 cals

Traditional Pork Goulash - 324 cals

Rainy Day Stew - 312 cals

Beef Bourguignon - 359 cals

Beef Burger and Sweet Potato Wedges - 353 cals

Beef Pot Roast - 390 cals

Beef With Mustard Sauce - 401 cals

Slow-Cooked Chilli Beef Stew - 401 cals

Sweet And Sour Pork - 493 cals

Sausage Cassoulet - 413 cals

Pork Stir-Fry With Noodles - 417 cals

Shepherds Pie - 479 cals

Zesty Pork Steaks With Mushrooms

224 calories

Serves 2 • Ready in 25 minutes

2 tsp sunflower oil (54 cals)
....
2 × 100g (3½oz) lean pork steaks (240 cals)
....
200g (7oz) mushrooms, sliced (26 cals)
....
1 heaped tsp paprika (14 cals)
....
1 tbsp cranberry jelly (24 cals)
....
zest and juice of 1 orange (52 cals)
....
1 tsp red wine vinegar (1 cal)
....
1 tsp (5g) butter (37 cals)
....

- Heat the oil in a large frying pan (skillet) over a medium-high heat. When hot, add the pork steaks and fry for 2 minutes on each side. At this stage the pork should be browned but not cooked through.

- Remove the pork from the pan and fry the mushrooms for about 5 minutes until soft.

- Return the pork to the pan and add the paprika, cranberry jelly, orange zest and juice and vinegar. Bring to a gentle simmer and stir to dissolve the cranberry jelly. Simmer for 5 minutes, turning the pork halfway through, until the meat is cooked.

- Remove the pork and mushrooms from the pan. Turn the heat up to medium and stir in the butter. Bubble for 2 minutes until the sauce is glossy.

Quick Italian Beef Stew

229 calories

Serves 2 • Ready in 30 minutes

1 tsp sunflower oil (27 cals)
....
200g (7oz) lean beef strips (246 cals)
....
salt and freshly ground black pepper
....
½ onion, peeled and sliced
into half rings (27 cals)
....
1 garlic clove, peeled and
thinly sliced (3 cals)
....
½ green (bell) pepper, deseeded
and sliced (10 cals)
....
½ yellow (bell) pepper, deseeded
and sliced (18 cals)
....
1 × 400g (14oz) can chopped
tomatoes (64 cals)
....
½ tsp dried mixed herbs
....
a little fresh oregano (optional)
....
12 large black olives, pitted (62 cals)
....

- Heat the oil in a large pan over a high heat. Season the beef with salt and pepper. When the oil is hot, toss in the beef and stir-fry for 2 minutes. Remove the beef from the pan and set aside.

- Reduce the heat to medium and fry the onion, garlic and (bell) peppers for 5–10 minutes until tender. With the heat still at medium, add the tomatoes and herbs and simmer for 15 minutes.

- Stir through the beef strips and olives and heat for a further 2 minutes before serving.

Asian-Style Stir-Fried Beef And Mushrooms

267 calories

Serves 2 • Ready in 15 minutes

2 tbsp dark soy sauce (9 cals)
juice of 1 lime (4 cals)
1 tsp sesame oil (30 cals)
½ tsp chilli (red pepper) flakes
200g (7oz) extra lean beef steak, cut into slivers (246 cals)
2 tsp sunflower oil (54 cals)
250g (9oz) mushrooms, sliced (32 cals)
1 × 300g (11oz) pack mixed vegetable stir-fry (158 cals)

- In a wide dish, mix together the soy sauce, lime juice, sesame oil and chilli flakes. Add the steak, turning to make sure all the pieces are fully covered. Cover the dish with clingfilm (plastic wrap) and leave to rest for at least 5 minutes.

- Heat the sunflower oil in a wok or wide frying pan (skillet) to a high temperature. Lift the beef from the marinade (setting the marinade aside for later) and stir-fry for 2 minutes until browned. Remove the meat from the wok and set aside.

- With the heat still on high, add the mushrooms and stir-fry for 2 minutes, then add the mixed veg and stir-fry for 1 more minute. Reduce the heat a little and return the beef to the pan. Pour over the rest of the marinade and toss everything together for 2 minutes until piping hot.

Minted Lamb with Butternut Crush

303 calories

Serves 2 • Ready in 30 minutes

300g (10½oz) (cut weight) butternut
squash, cubed (96 cals)

1 tsp olive oil (27 cals)

1 garlic clove, peeled (4 cals)

salt and freshly ground black pepper

2 fresh mint leaves

large bunch of flat-leaf
(Italian) parsley (3 cals)

juice of 1 lemon (3 cals)

2 tbsp extra virgin olive oil (198 cals)

2 × 90g (3¼oz) lean lamb
leg steaks (275 cals)

- Preheat the oven to 220C/200C Fan/425F.

- Arrange the butternut squash over a baking tray and drizzle a teaspoon of olive oil over the top. Bake in the oven for 20 minutes.

- Meanwhile, place the garlic, a little salt, the herbs and lemon juice in a blender and process until they form a paste. If you don't have a blender, you can chop the ingredients finely instead. Gradually pour in the olive oil, blending until it forms a smooth emulsified sauce. Transfer the sauce to a wide dish that is big enough to hold the lamb.

- Preheat the grill (broiler) to medium-high. Season the lamb and place under the grill. Cook for 5–8 minutes on each side, depending on how you like your lamb. It should be seared on the outside and if you like it a little pink, you should make sure the inside gets properly hot – 145°C/293°F on a meat thermometer.

- Transfer the lamb to the serving dish and scoop up the sauce over the top. Leave to rest in the sauce for a few minutes before serving.

- Remove the butternut from the oven and use the back of a fork to lightly crush. Divide between two plates and arrange the lamb over the top.

Lamb Tagine

303 calories

Serves 4 • Ready in 2 hours

1 tbsp vegetable oil (99 cals)

1 tbsp plain (all-purpose) flour, seasoned with salt and freshly ground black pepper (68 cals)

300g (11oz) extra lean lamb, diced (459 cals)

1 medium onion, chopped (54 cals)

2 tsp mild chilli powder

1 tsp turmeric

1 tsp ground cumin

1 × 400g (14oz) can chopped tomatoes (64 cals)

500ml (generous 2 cups) lamb/ chicken or vegetable stock (made with 1 cube) (35 cals)

100g (½ cup) pearl barley (360 cals)

1 tbsp shop-bought salsa (7 cals)

1 tbsp apricot jam (63 cals)

juice of 1 lime (4 cals)

- Preheat the oven to 180C/160C fan/350F if using. Heat the oil in a large lidded casserole dish over a high heat.

- Sprinkle the seasoned flour over the diced lamb and use your hands to mix it through and make sure all the surfaces of the meat are covered.

- When the oil is hot, toss in the meat and fry for about 2 minutes without stirring. Then stir, turn and fry the other side for a further 2 minutes. Remove the lamb from the dish with a slotted spoon.

- Turn the heat down to low and add the onion. Stir in the spices, then add the chopped tomatoes and stock. Bring to the boil. Add the pearl barley and boil vigorously for 10 minutes.
- Return the lamb to the casserole. Stir in the salsa, jam and lime juice. Put the lid on and cook in the oven for 2 hours OR transfer to a slow cooker and cook on low for 6–8 hours.

Grilled Lamb With Tangy Lemon Couscous

314 calories

Serves 2 • Ready in 30 minutes

1 tsp olive oil (27 cals)

1 garlic clove, peeled and
finely sliced (3 cals)

100g (½ cup) couscous (dried
weight) (227 cals)

250ml (generous 1 cup) hot chicken
stock (made with ½ cube) (17 cals)

2 × 90g (3¼oz) lean lamb
leg steaks (337 cals)

salt and freshly ground black pepper

zest and juice of 1 lemon (4 cals)

50g (1¾oz) rocket (arugula) (13 cals)

- Heat the oil in a medium lidded saucepan over a medium heat. Add the garlic and fry for about 2 minutes or until golden, then stir in the couscous. Fry the couscous for 1–2 minutes, stirring constantly. Turn the heat off.

- Add the hot stock to the couscous and stir gently. Put the lid on the pan and leave the couscous to 'cook' for about 15 minutes. When cooked all the liquid will have been absorbed and the couscous will be tender with just a little bite.

- While the couscous is cooking, heat the grill (broiler) to a medium-high setting.

- Season the lamb with salt and pepper and place under the hot grill. The cooking time will depend on thickness and desired degree of doneness. Anything from 5–8 minutes on each side. If you have a meat thermometer the internal temp should reach 145C/293F.

- Set the lamb aside and cover for 5 minutes. Resting makes the meat more tender.

- When both the lamb and couscous are done, stir the lemon zest and juice of half the lemon into the couscous, then stir in the rocket (arugula).

- Serve with the lamb resting on top of the couscous and squeezing on a little of the remaining lemon juice.

Traditional Pork Goulash

324 calories

Serves 4 • Ready in 2 hours

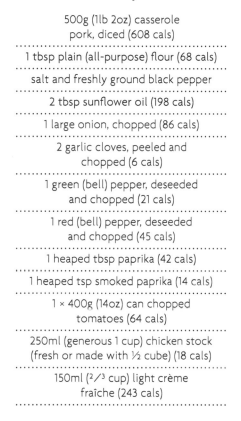

500g (1lb 2oz) casserole
pork, diced (608 cals)
....
1 tbsp plain (all-purpose) flour (68 cals)
....
salt and freshly ground black pepper
....
2 tbsp sunflower oil (198 cals)
....
1 large onion, chopped (86 cals)
....
2 garlic cloves, peeled and
chopped (6 cals)
....
1 green (bell) pepper, deseeded
and chopped (21 cals)
....
1 red (bell) pepper, deseeded
and chopped (45 cals)
....
1 heaped tbsp paprika (42 cals)
....
1 heaped tsp smoked paprika (14 cals)
....
1 × 400g (14oz) can chopped
tomatoes (64 cals)
....
250ml (generous 1 cup) chicken stock
(fresh or made with ½ cube) (18 cals)
....
150ml (²⁄³ cup) light crème
fraîche (243 cals)
....

- Sprinkle the pork with the flour and salt and pepper and toss until well coated.

- Heat the oil in a casserole dish over a high heat. Brown the pork in batches and set aside.

- Turn the heat to low and add the onion, garlic and (bell) peppers. Put the lid on and sweat until tender, about 10 minutes.

- Return the pork to the pan together with both types of paprika, the chopped tomatoes and stock. Bring to a simmer and cook with the lid off for 20–30 minutes.

On the hob

- Continue to cook over a low heat for about 1 hour, removing the lid towards the end of the cooking time.

In the oven

- Preheat the oven to 150C/130C fan/300F and cook for 3 hours.

In the slow cooker

- Transfer to a slow cooker and cook on low for 8 hours or overnight. Stir in the crème fraîche just before serving. The goulash freezes well and this can be done before or after the crème fraîche is added.

Rainy Day Stew

337 calories

Serves 2 • Ready in 45 minutes

1 litre (4 cups) chicken stock
(fresh is best here) (70 cals)

1 leek, trimmed and sliced (26 cals)

2 good quality pork sausages, sliced
into 2cm (¾in) pieces (256 cals)

1 red chilli, deseeded if preferred
and sliced (4 cals)

2 bay leaves

½ tsp dried mixed herbs or small handful
of fresh basil and/or parsley if available

1 courgette (zucchini), halved
and sliced (27 cals)

50g (scant ½ cup) peas, fresh
or frozen (42 cals)

50g (1¾oz) chonchigliette (or
other small pasta) (174 cals)

2 medium tomatoes, diced (29 cals)

salt and freshly ground black pepper

10g (2 tbsp) fresh Parmesan,
grated (45 cals)

- Heat the chicken stock in a large saucepan with the leek, sausages, chilli, bay leaves and dried herbs. Bring to a gentle simmer and cook for about 25 minutes.

- Add the courgette (zucchini), peas and macaroni and simmer for a further 10–15 minutes until the pasta and peas are tender.

- Remove the bay leaves from the pan and add the tomatoes and any fresh herbs if using.

- Serve in large bowls and season generously. Sprinkle the grated Parmesan over the top.

Beef Bourguignon

359 calories

Serves 4 • Ready in 3 hours

400g (14oz) extra lean casserole
beef steak, diced (492 cals)

....

100g (3½oz) lardons or
bacon bits (276 cals)

....

200g (7oz) button mushrooms,
washed (26 cals)

....

2 garlic cloves, peeled and sliced (6 cals)

....

1 medium onion, peeled,
halved and sliced (54 cals)

....

200g (7oz) pickled shallots,
drained (30 cals)

....

1 tsp dried thyme (3 cals)

....

2 bay leaves

....

2 tbsp plain (all-purpose) flour (204 cals)

....

salt and freshly ground black pepper

....

400ml (1¾ cups) red wine (344 cals)

....

- Put the beef, lardons, mushrooms, garlic, onion, shallots, thyme and bay leaves into a large casserole dish or slow cooker dish.

- Sprinkle on the flour and, using your hands, toss it around until everything is lightly coated in flour. Next, season with salt and pepper and pour on the wine and 100ml (scant ½ cup) water. Give it a stir and pop on the lid.

In the oven

- Preheat the oven to 140C/120C fan/275F and cook for 3 hours.

In the slow cooker

- Cook on low for 8 hrs. Add a little water halfway through cooking if necessary.

Homemade Beef Burger and Sweet Potato Wedges

353 calories

Serves 2 • Ready in 45 minutes

200g sweet potatoes (2 small)
(174 cals including skin)

....

salt and freshly ground black pepper

....

2 tsp sunflower oil (54 cals)

....

250g (9oz) extra-lean minced
(ground) beef (435 cals)

....

2 spring onions (scallions) (10 cals)

....

1 small garlic clove, peeled and
finely chopped (3 cals)

....

½ tsp dried herbs

....

1 tsp Worcestershire sauce (3 cals)

....

salt and freshly ground black pepper

....

1 tsp olive oil (27 cals)

....

- Preheat the oven to 220C/200C fan/425F.

- Peel and cut the sweet potatoes into large wedges. If you prefer you can leave the skin on the potatoes.

- Place the sweet potato wedges into a pan of cold, salted water and bring to the boil. Cook for 15 minutes from cold. Drain and leave to cool until they are cold enough to handle.

- Place the sweet potatoes in a roasting tray and pour on the oil. Toss through with your hands so that the potatoes are as covered as possible and season well. Bake in the oven for 25–30 minutes until crispy and golden.

- Place the beef, spring onions (scallions), garlic, dried herbs, Worcestershire sauce and salt and pepper in a large bowl and mix together by hand until fully combined. Divide the mixture into 4 equal pieces and roll each one into a ball, then flatten with the palm of your hand to make a burger shape. Place the burgers on a plate, cover and chill in the refrigerator for half an hour (or in the freezer for 10 minutes).

- Heat the olive oil in a wide frying pan (skillet) and fry for 8–10 minutes, turning once. Serve immediately.

Beef Pot Roast

390 calories

Serves 4 • Ready in 2 hours 30 minutes

450g extra lean casserole beef
steak, diced (765 cals)

2 tsp turmeric

2 tsp English mustard (22 cals)

1 tsp sugar (16 cals)

salt and freshly ground black pepper

1 tbsp vegetable oil (99 cals)

1 medium onion, peeled
and chopped (54 cals)

4 garlic cloves, peeled and
chopped (12 cals)

1 medium sweet potato (about 130g),
peeled and cut into large chunks (113 cals)

1 × 400g (14oz) can whole
tomatoes (64 cals)

1 × 400g (14oz) can chickpeas,
rinsed and drained (276 cals)

500ml (generous 2 cups) beef or chicken
stock (made from 1 stock cube) (35 cals)

100g (3½oz) spinach, fresh or
frozen (about 4 cubes) (21 cals)

100g (scant 1 cup) peas, fresh (83 cals)

- Rub the beef all over with the turmeric, mustard, sugar and salt and pepper.

- In a casserole dish, heat the vegetable oil until it is smoking hot. Toss in the beef and fry for 2 minutes each side. Reduce the heat and stir in the onion and garlic and fry gently for 2 minutes.

- Add the sweet potato, tomatoes, chickpeas and stock, then stir and put the lid on.

In the oven

- Preheat the oven to 180C/160C fan/350F and cook for 2 hours.
- Stir in the spinach and peas. Replace onto the hob, bring to a gentle simmer and cook for 10 minutes.

In the slow cooker

- Cook on low for 7–8 hours. Stir in the spinach and peas.
- Turn to high and cook uncovered for 30 minutes.

Beef With Mustard Sauce

401 calories

Serves 1 • Ready in 20 minutes

150g (5oz) new potatoes (about 3
med), with skin on, halved (105 cals)

....

½ tsp olive oil (14 cals)

....

150g (5oz) extra-lean beef
escalope (scallop) (184 cals)

....

1 tsp roughly ground black pepper

....

a pinch of salt

....

For the mustard sauce:

....

½ tsp olive oil (14 cals)

....

½ shallot, peeled and very
finely diced (3 cals)

....

1 tbsp brandy (31 cals)

....

½ tsp English mustard (3 cals)

....

1 tsp Dijon mustard (7 cals)

....

1 tbsp light crème fraîche (40 cals)

....

- Cook the potatoes in boiling water for 15-20 minutes.

- Rub a little olive oil over both sides of the steak. Sprinkle the roughly ground pepper on a plate with the salt, add the steak and turn until it is coated on all sides with the pepper. Leave to rest for at least 5 minutes.

- Heat a frying pan (skillet) over a very high heat. When the pan is properly hot, add the peppered steak and cook for 2–4 minutes on each side, depending on thickness and how you like your steak cooked. Don't overcook as the meat will become tough. When cooked, cover and leave to rest for 5 minutes while you finish the mustard sauce.

- To make the sauce, heat the olive oil in a small frying pan over a low heat and toss in the diced shallot. Cook gently for 5–10 minutes until translucent. Increase the heat to medium, add the brandy and let it bubble for 1 minute before reducing the heat again. Add both mustards and the crème fraîche, stir well and cook for a further 2 minutes.

- Place the potatoes and steak on a serving plate and pour the sauce over to serve.

Slow-Cooked Chilli Beef Stew

401 calories

Serves 4 • Ready in 1 hour

2 tsp sunflower oil (54 cals)

1 large onion, peeled and
chopped (90 cals)

2 fresh green or red chillies, deseeded
and chopped into rings (3 cals)

2 garlic cloves, peeled and
roughly chopped (6 cals)

450g (1lb) extra-lean casserole
beef steak, diced (581 cals)

1 tsp mild chilli powder

1 tsp ground cumin

2 tsp paprika (14 cals)

1 tsp salt

1 tsp cocoa powder (unsweetened
cocoa) (6 cals)

juice of 1 lime (3 cals)

1 × 400g (14oz) can chopped
tomatoes (64 cals)

1 × 400g (14oz) can red kidney beans,
drained and rinsed (210 cals)

160g (¾ cup) basmati rice (574 cals)

- Heat the oil in a large casserole over a medium heat, add the onion and gently fry for about 5 minutes. Add the chillies and garlic and fry for a further 2 minutes.

- Using a slotted spoon, remove the onion, chillies and garlic from the pan and turn the heat to high. Add the beef to the pan in 2 batches and fry until browned on all sides.

- Reduce the heat, return all the meat to the pan, together with the onion mixture and stir in the chilli powder, cumin, paprika, salt and cocoa. Finally, add the lime juice, canned tomatoes and kidney beans and stir well. Bring to the boil, reduce the heat and simmer gently for 30–40 minutes, stirring occasionally.

- Alternatively, transfer to a slow cooker and cook on low for about 8 hours or cook in a lidded casserole in an oven preheated to 160C/fan 140C/325F for 2 hours.

- Cook the rice according to your preferred method.

Sweet And Sour Pork

493 calories

Serves 2 • Ready in 15 minutes

80g (3oz) basmati rice (282 cals)
....
1 × 175g (6oz) lean pork tenderloin
fillet, thinly sliced (394 cals)
....
½ level tbsp plain (all-purpose)
flour, seasoned with salt and freshly
ground black pepper (34 cals)
....
2 tsp olive oil (54 cals)
....
1 garlic clove, peeled and
finely chopped (3 cals)
....
4 spring onions (scallions), trimmed
and shredded (18 cals)
....
½ red (bell) pepper, deseeded
and finely sliced (26 cals)
....
½ yellow (bell) pepper, deseeded
and finely sliced (21 cals)
....
1 x 200g (7oz) can pineapple
chunks in juice (126 cals)
....
1 tbsp white wine vinegar (3 cals)
....
1 tsp tomato purée (paste) (8 cals)
....
1 tbsp light soy sauce (4 cals)
....
1 tbsp dry sherry (14 cals)
....

- Cook the rice by your preferred method.

- Toss the pork in the seasoned flour until lightly coated.

- Heat the olive oil in a wide saucepan or wok over a medium-high heat. Add the pork and stir-fry until just cooked, about 4–5 minutes. Remove the pork from the pan with a slotted spoon, cover and keep warm.

- Return the pan to a medium heat, add the garlic and spring onions (scallions) and stir-fry for 1 minute before adding the (bell) peppers and stir-frying for a further 3 minutes.
- Return the pork to the pan. Stir in the pineapple chunks and about 2 tbsp of their juice. Then add the vinegar, tomato purée (paste), soy sauce, water and the sherry. Simmer for 2 more minutes before serving over the rice.

Sausage Cassoulet

413 calories

Serves 4 • Ready in 1 hour

1 tsp olive oil (27 cals)
4 sausages (662 cals)
1 onion, finely chopped (65 cals)
2 cloves garlic, chopped (6 cals)
1 carrot, diced (35 cals)
1 red (bell) pepper, diced (54 cals)
1 green (bell) pepper, diced (26 cals)
200g (1 cup) red lentils (678 cals)
1 litre (4 cups) water
1 chicken stock cube (35 cals)
1 bay leaf
1 x 400g (14oz) can chopped tomatoes (64 cals)

- In a heavy based lidded saucepan, heat the oil at a medium temperature and fry the sausages until they are tinged with brown. Remove the sausages from the pan and set aside.

- Turn the heat to low and add the onion, garlic, carrot and peppers. Stir and leave to saute gently for 5 minutes.

- Next, add in the lentils and mix into the vegetables. Then pour in the water, turn the heat to high and bring to the boil. Crumble the stock cube into the pan and add the bay leaf too. When the lentils start to boil, turn the heat to medium (bubbling vigorously) and cook for 10 minutes.

- After 10 minutes turn the heat to low, add the tomatoes and stir. Then put the sausages into the top of the pan and put the lid on. Cook on the lowest heat possible for 45 minutes to 1 hour. Alternatively, transfer the pan to the oven and cook at 180C/160C Fan/360F for 45 minutes to 1 hour.

Pork Stir-Fry With Noodles

417 calories

Serves 2 • Ready in 15 minutes

1 tsp sunflower oil (27 cals)

½ onion, peeled and finely
chopped (32 cals)

½ red (bell) pepper, deseeded
and cut into strips (26 cals)

160g (5½oz) lean pork tenderloin,
cut into thin strips (394 cals)

1 red chilli, deseeded and
cut into rings (3 cals)

1 garlic clove, peeled and
finely chopped (3 cals)

1 × 225g (8oz) can water chestnuts,
drained and sliced (70 cals)

200g (7oz) fresh rice noodles (256 cals)

1 tbsp dark soy sauce (4 cals)

½ tbsp mirin (rice wine) or sherry (18 cals)

- • Heat the oil in a wok or wide saucepan over a medium-high heat, add the onion and red (bell) pepper and stir-fry for 3 minutes. Add the pork, chilli and garlic and stir-fry for a further 3 minutes. Add the water chestnuts and cook for 2 minutes.

- • Add the noodles to the stir-fry. Blend the soy sauce and mirin (rice wine) or sherry together in a small bowl, then mix into the stir-fry. Cook for a further 2 minutes, then serve.

Shepherds Pie

479 calories

You can make a similar dish using minced (ground) beef and call it Cottage Pie.

Serves 4 • Ready in 1 hour 30 minutes

1 tbsp olive oil (99 cals)

1 medium onion, peeled
and chopped (54 cals)

4 garlic cloves, peeled and
chopped (12 cals)

500g (1lb 2oz) 10% fat minced
(ground) lamb (756 cals)

1 tsp turmeric

2 tsp English mustard (22 cals)

1 tbsp ketchup (29 cals)

salt and freshly ground black pepper

100g (½ cup) red lentils (353 cals)

500ml (generous 2 cups) lamb or chicken
stock (made from 1 stock cube) (35 cals)

100g (3½oz) spinach, fresh or
frozen(about 4 cubes) (21 cals)

100g (scant 1 cup) peas, fresh (83 cals)

500g (1lb 2oz) sweet potato (about 4 med),
peeled and cut into large chunks (452 cals)

- Preheat the oven to 180C/160C fan/350F.

- In a large saucepan, heat the oil and gently fry the onion and garlic for 5 minutes.

- Turn the heat up a little and add the lamb mince. Fry until browned, breaking up bigger pieces of mince with the back of a wooden spoon. Stir in the turmeric, mustard, ketchup and season generously with salt and pepper.

- Add the lentils and stock and simmer for 15 minutes.
- Meanwhile, boil the sweet potatoes for 15 minutes until soft. Then mash.
- Add the spinach and peas to the lamb. Remove from the heat and transfer to a baking dish. Scoop the sweet potato over the lamb and spread evenly with the back of a fork.
- Bake in the oven for 1 hour.

Veggie

Leek And Olive Pasta - 233 cals

Asparagus and Cherry Tomato Pasta - 260 cals

Mixed Bean Chilli - 267 cals

Vegetarian Bolognaise - 292 cals

Multi-Coloured Pepper Bake - 293 cals

East African Vegetable Curry - 262 cals

Spinach & Pea Rice With Paneer - 298 cals

Vegetarian Curry Pot - 300 cals

Bean Burgers, New Pots & Mange Tout - 303 cals

Baked Mushroom & Blue Cheese Risotto - 304 cals

Parsnip And Leek Frittata - 348 cals

Autumn Vegetable Bake - 321 cals

Leek And Olive Pasta

233 calories

Serves 1 • Ready in 15 minutes

50g (2oz) penne pasta (177 cals)

1 tsp olive oil (27 cals)

2 leeks, trimmed and cut into
1cm (½in) wide slices (52 cals)

zest of 1 lemon

juice of ½ lemon (2 cals)

1 tsp extra virgin olive oil (27 cals)

salt and freshly ground black pepper

10g (2 tbsp) Parmesan, fresh
grated (83 cals)

50g (1¾oz) watercress or baby
spinach leaves (11 cals)

6 black olives, pitted (31 cals)

- Cook the pasta in boiling water, according to the pack instructions.

- In a wide lidded pan, heat the olive oil over a medium-high heat. When hot, add the leeks and stir-fry for 2 minutes. Reduce the heat, add about 2 tablespoons water and put the lid on. Steam until tender, about 10 minutes.

- Combine the lemon zest, lemon juice, extra virgin olive oil, salt and pepper and half the Parmesan in a small bowl.

- Stir the watercress, olives and lemon dressing through the leeks and pasta.

- Transfer to a serving bowl and sprinkle on the remaining Parmesan. Season generously with salt and pepper and serve.

Asparagus and Cherry Tomato Pasta

260 calories

Serves 1 • Ready in 15 minutes

50g (2oz) conchiglie (shell) pasta (177 cals)

100g (3½oz) fine asparagus, chopped (25 cals)

10 cherry tomatoes, quartered (22 cals)

2 spring onions (scallions), trimmed and chopped (10 cals)

1 tsp extra virgin olive oil (27 cals)

1 tsp balsamic vinegar (5 cals)

1 slice Parma ham (prosciutto), cut into pieces (27 cals)

5g (1 tsp) Parmesan cheese, finely grated (21 cals)

salt and freshly ground black pepper

- Cook the pasta according to instructions.
- Lightly cook the asparagus by plunging into boiling water and boiling for 4–5 minutes, until just tender.
- Mix together the cherry tomatoes with the spring onions, olive oil and balsamic vinegar.
- Combine the pasta and asparagus in a bowl and pour the cherry tomatoes over. Finally, sprinkle on the Parmesan cheese and a generous seasoning of salt and pepper.

Mixed Bean Chilli

267 calories

Serves 4 • Ready in 1 hour 30 minutes

1 tsp olive oil (27 cals)

1 medium onion, peeled
and chopped (54 cals)

1 green chilli, deseeded and
finely chopped (1 cal)

1 red (bell) pepper, deseeded
and finely chopped (45 cals)

2 garlic cloves, peeled and
thinly sliced (6 cals)

¼ tsp chilli (red pepper) flakes

1 tsp mild chilli powder

½ tsp ground cumin

1 heaped tsp paprika (14 cals)

½ tsp (unsweetened) cocoa
powder (3 cals)

salt and freshly ground black pepper

1kg (2.2lb) (cut weight) butternut
squash, cubed (380 cals)

1 × 400g (14oz) can chopped
tomatoes (64 cals)

1 × 400g (14oz) can kidney beans,
rinsed and drained (210 cals)

1 × 400g (14oz) can cannellini beans,
rinsed and drained (259 cals)

juice of 1 lime (4 cals)

- In a large lidded casserole, heat the oil gently and add the onion, chilli, red (bell) pepper and garlic. Sweat gently with the lid on for about 10–15 minutes until tender.

- Add the spices, cocoa and salt and pepper and stir. Add the butternut squash and stir again.
- Next pour in the chopped tomatoes, both types of beans and top up with 400ml (1¾ cups) water – making sure all the ingredients are generously covered with the water.
- Bring to a simmer, cover and cook slowly for 1 hour.
- If you prefer you could cook in the oven at 190C/170C fan/375F for 1 hour or in the slow cooker on low for 6–8 hours.
- Crush some of the butternut squash and/or beans with the back of the spoon to thicken the sauce. Stir in the lime juice and season to taste before serving.

Vegetarian Bolognaise

292 calories

Note: If you can't get hold of paneer, drained & crumbled ricotta works well. A vegan alternative would be a firm tofu, crumbled.

Serves 6 • Ready in 1 hour 30 minutes

2 tbsp olive oil (198 cals)

1 large onion, chopped (86 cals)

4 cloves garlic, peeled and sliced (15 cals)

1 carrot, peeled and chopped (35 cals)

2 celery sticks, trimmed
and chopped (10 cals)

1 green (bell) pepper, seeded
and chopped (24 cals)

1 courgette (zucchini), trimmed
and chopped (27 cals)

180g (6½oz) dried red lentils (572 cals)

250ml (1 cup) water

2 x 400g (14oz) tin chopped
tomatoes (128 cals)

1 bay leaf

½ tsp chilli flakes

1 tsp tamarind paste (12 cals)

1 tbsp cider vinegar (4 cals)

1 tbsp tomato ketchup (29 cals)

1 tbsp tomato paste (30 cals)

1 tsp salt

1 heaped tsp dark brown sugar (32 cals)

200g (7oz) paneer, finely chopped
and crumbled (348 cals)

200ml (generous ¾ cup) red wine (172 cals)

250g (9oz) mushrooms, washed
and sliced (32 cals)

··

- In a large pan, heat the oil over a medium heat. Fry the onion for 5 minutes. Add the garlic, carrot, celery, green pepper and courgette (zucchini). Cook for 10 minutes until soft, stirring frequently. Stir in the lentils, then add the water and chopped tomatoes. Bring to the boil and cook on a vigorous heat for 10 minutes.

- Reduce the heat to medium/low, add the bay leaf, chilli flakes, tamarind, vinegar, ketchup, tomato paste, salt and sugar. Crumble in the paneer (the smaller the better) and add the wine and mushrooms. Cook for a further 30 minutes to an hour until the sauce is rich and thick.

Multi-Coloured Pepper Bake

293 calories

Serves 4 • Ready in 1 hour

1 tsp olive oil (27 cals)

....

1 large onion, peeled and
finely chopped (72 cals)

....

1 garlic clove, peeled and
finely chopped (3 cals)

....

100g (3½oz) dried Puy (French
green) lentils (297 cals)

....

1 vegetable stock cube (33 cals)

....

4 red (bell) peppers, deseeded
and chopped (205 cals)

....

2 yellow (bell) peppers, deseeded
and chopped (84 cals)

....

2 green (bell) peppers, deseeded
and chopped (48 cals)

....

1 large cooking apple, peeled,
cored and chopped (80 cals)

....

2 tsp dried basil (3 cals)

....

50ml (scant ¼ cup) white wine (33 cals)

....

1 × 400g (14oz) can chopped
tomatoes (64 cals)

....

25g (1oz) mature (sharp) Cheddar
cheese, grated (104 cals)

....

10g (1/3oz) Parmesan cheese,
finely grated (45 cals)

....

20g panko breadcrumbs (75 cals)

....

- Preheat the oven to 180C/fan 160C/350F.

- Heat the olive oil gently in a large saucepan, add the onion and garlic and fry for 5 minutes or until the onion turns translucent.

Add the lentils, stir, then add 600ml (2½ cups) water and crumble in the stock cube. Bring to the boil, then reduce the heat and simmer for 25 minutes.

- Next, add all the peppers, apple, basil, white wine and canned tomatoes and mix well.
- Transfer the mixture to an ovenproof baking dish and sprinkle the 2 grated cheeses and the breadcrumbs over the top. Cook in the oven for 30 minutes. Serve immediately or cool and freeze in individual portions.

East African Vegetable Curry

262 calories

Serves 2 • Ready in 45 minutes

1 tsp olive oil (27 cals)

1 onion, peeled and chopped (54 cals)

1 garlic clove, finely chopped (3 cals)

2 tsp ground cumin

¼ tsp ground cinnamon

2 tsp ground coriander

1 tbsp tomato purée (paste) (30 cals)

1 tsp harissa paste (4 cals)

½ red (bell) pepper, diced (27 cals)

1 × 200g (7oz) can chickpeas
(or half 400g/14oz can), rinsed
and drained (138 cals)

40g (scant ¼ cup) red lentils (dry
weight), rinsed (127 cals)

1 potato (170g/6oz), peeled
and diced (75 cals)

500ml (generous 2 cups) vegetable stock
(fresh or made with 1 cube) (35 cals)

juice of 1 lemon (3 cals)

- Heat the oil in a large saucepan, add the onion and fry for 7–8 minutes until translucent. Add the garlic and fry for 1 more minute. Stir in the spices, tomato purée (paste) and harissa paste, then add the diced pepper and fry for 3 minutes.

- Add the chickpeas, lentils, potato, stock and lemon juice. Bring to the boil, reduce the heat slightly and simmer vigorously for 10 minutes, before reducing the heat and simmering gently for a further 15 minutes.

Spinach & Pea Rice With Paneer

298 calories

If you can't get hold of paneer, the best substitute for this recipe would be queso blanco.

Serves 2 • Ready in 45 minutes

80g (3oz) brown rice, rinsed (286 cals)
1 tbsp sunflower oil (99 cals)
1 onion, peeled and chopped (54 cals)
1 bird's eye (Thai) chilli, deseeded and finely chopped (1 cal)
½ tsp aniseed seeds (optional)
½ tsp garam masala
½ tsp ground cumin
a pinch of salt
100g (3½oz) frozen spinach, defrosted (21 cals)
80g (3oz) frozen peas (52 cals)
200g (7oz) paneer, roughly chopped (348 cals)
1 handful of fresh coriander (cilantro), chopped (3 cals)
juice of ½ lemon (2 cals)

- Cook the brown rice in a pan of boiling water for about 35–40 minutes, or according to the packet instructions. Drain.

- Heat the oil in a wide frying pan (skillet) over a medium heat. Add the onion, chilli and aniseed (if using), then stir, reduce the heat and cook for 5–10 minutes until the onion is translucent.

- Add the ground spices and salt to the pan. Stir for 30 seconds. Add the spinach, peas and paneer and increase the heat to medium. Stir-fry for 2–3 minutes, then add the cooked rice, coriander (cilantro) and lemon juice. Stir–fry for a further minute until everything is mixed and the rice is warm.

Vegetarian Curry Pot

300 calories

If you can't get hold of paneer, the best substitute for this recipe would be queso blanco.

Serves 4 • Ready in 1 hour

1 tbsp olive oil (99 cals)

1 large onion, peeled and
finely chopped (86 cals)

4 garlic cloves, peeled and
finely chopped (12 cals)

2.5cm (1in) piece fresh root ginger,
peeled and grated (5 cals)

1 large red chilli, deseeded and
chopped into fine rings (3 cals)

¼ tsp ground turmeric

¼ tsp cayenne pepper

1 tsp paprika (7 cals)

½ tsp ground cumin

a pinch of salt

180g (6½oz) dried red lentils,
rinsed (572 cals)

200g paneer, roughly chopped (348 cals)

juice of 2 limes (7 cals)

1 tomato, finely chopped (14 cals)

75g (3oz) frozen peas (50 cals)

- Heat the oil in a heavy-based pan over a low-medium heat. Add the onion, garlic, ginger and chilli and stir-fry for 3–4 minutes. Add the ground spices and salt and stir-fry for another minute. Add the lentils, stir, then pour in 900ml (3½ cups) water and bring to the boil.

- Reduce the heat slightly and simmer vigorously for 10 minutes.

- Reduce the heat to low and cook for a further 30-40 minutes, stirring regularly, until all the water has been absorbed. If the dal is too thick or starts to stick on the base of the pan, just add a little more water.

- When the dal has the consistency of thick porridge, add the paneer, lime juice and tomato and cook for a further 5 minutes before serving.

Bean Burgers With New Potatoes And Mange Tout

303 calories

Serves 2 • Ready in 20 minutes

200g (7oz) new potatoes (about 4 med), with skin on, quartered (140 cals)

200g (7oz) mange tout (snow peas), trimmed (74 cals)

1 × 400g (14oz) can cannellini beans, rinsed and drained (259 cals)

1 tsp tomato purée (paste) (8 cals)

1 heaped tsp cornflour (cornstarch) (15 cals)

2 spring onions (scallions), trimmed and chopped (10 cals)

1 clove garlic, peeled and crushed (4 cals)

1 tsp mild chilli powder

¼ tsp ground turmeric

Salt and freshly ground black pepper

1 tsp mayonnaise (33 cals)

1 tbsp natural yogurt (22 cals)

1 tbsp rice wine (3 cals)

2 fresh mint leaves, finely chopped

2 spring onions (scallions), trimmed and sliced (10 cals)

1 tsp olive oil (27 cals)

• Quarter the potatoes and steam or boil until tender. Add the mange tout (snow peas) for the last 4-5 minutes of cooking time. Drain and cover.

- Place the beans in a large bowl and use a potato masher or fork to thoroughly mash the beans. Add the tomato purée, cornflour, spring onion, garlic, chilli powder and turmeric. Season generously with salt and pepper. Mix well.

- Divide the mixture into four portions and form into balls, then flatten a little to form a burger. If you have time, chill for 30 minutes or freeze for 10 minutes. The burgers will hold their shape slightly better if chilled but will be just as delicious if cooked straight away.

- In a small bowl, combine the mayonnaise, yogurt, rice wine, mint leaves and spring onions. Leave for 5-10 minutes for the flavours to develop.

- Heat the oil in a frying pan over a medium heat. Add the burgers to the pan and cook for 3–4 minutes on one side. Turn with a fish slice and flatten a little more if necessary. Cook for a further 3–4 minutes until golden brown.

- Arrange the warm potatoes and mange tout over two plates. Place the burgers on the top. Finally pour over the dressing. Serve immediately.

Baked Mushroom And Blue Cheese Risotto

304 calories

Serves 2 • Ready in 1 hour

1 tsp olive oil (27 cals)

1 red onion, peeled and chopped (54 cals)

200g (7oz) mushrooms, sliced (26 cals)

100g (½ cup) brown rice, rinsed (357 cals)

300ml (1¼ cups) vegetable stock (fresh or made with ½ cube) (18 cals)

juice of ½ lemon (2 cals)

30g (scant ¼ cup) blue cheese, crumbled (123 cals)

salt and freshly ground black pepper

- Preheat the oven to 200C/180C fan/400F.

- Heat the oil in an ovenproof casserole, add the onion and fry for 3 minutes. Toss in the mushrooms and fry for a further 2 minutes.

- Tip in the rice and stir through. Add the stock and bring to a gentle simmer.

- Cover with a lid and place in the oven. Cook for 45–55 minutes (reduce this to 20 minutes if you are using white rice), checking if you need to add more water halfway through, until the rice is tender.

- Stir through the lemon juice and blue cheese. Season to taste before serving.

Parsnip And Leek Frittata

348 calories

Serves 2 • Ready in 30 minutes

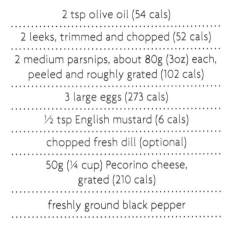

2 tsp olive oil (54 cals)

2 leeks, trimmed and chopped (52 cals)

2 medium parsnips, about 80g (3oz) each,
peeled and roughly grated (102 cals)

3 large eggs (273 cals)

½ tsp English mustard (6 cals)

chopped fresh dill (optional)

50g (¼ cup) Pecorino cheese,
grated (210 cals)

freshly ground black pepper

- In a lidded frying pan (skillet) heat half the oil over a medium–high heat. Toss in the leeks & grated parsnips and stir-fry for 2 minutes. Reduce the heat, add 2 tablespoons water & put the lid on. Sweat the leeks and parsnips for 10 minutes. Leave to cool.

- Put the eggs, mustard and dill in a bowl and whisk thoroughly. Stir in the grated cheese and cooled vegetables.

- Preheat the grill (broiler) to a medium setting.

- Choose a frying pan with a metal handle that can go under the grill. Wipe with kitchen paper (paper towels) dipped in the remaining oil. Heat over a medium–high heat and, when hot, add the egg mixture. Roll the pan around so the egg covers the base of the pan evenly. Immediately turn the heat to the lowest setting and cook, uncovered, for about 10 minutes or until the base and sides are firm.

- Sprinkle over the black pepper and put the pan under the grill for another 5–10 minutes until the top is firm and golden.

- Invert onto a plate. Serve immediately or leave to cool and serve in wedges.

Autumn Vegetable Bake

321 calories

Serves 4 • Ready in 1 hour 30 minutes

2 tbsp olive oil (198 cals)

1 large onion, peeled and chopped (86 cals)

2 garlic cloves, peeled and sliced (6 cals)

1 red chilli, deseeded and chopped (3 cals)

1 × 400g (14oz) can chopped tomatoes (64 cals)

300ml (1¼ cups) white wine (198 cals)

500ml (generous 2 cups) vegetable stock (35 cals)

1 bay leaf

2 fresh thyme sprigs (or ½ tsp dried)

500g (1lb 2oz) (cut weight) butternut squash, cubed (190 cals)

1 × 400g (14oz) can butter (lima) beans, rinsed and drained (220 cals)

50g (1/3 cup) wholemeal (wholewheat) breadcrumbs (108 cals)

5g (1 tsp) Parmesan, grated (21 cals)

25g (1 oz) chopped nuts (152 cals)

handful of fresh parsley, chopped (3 cals)

Salt and freshly ground black pepper

- Heat 1 tablespoon of oil in a large pan, add the onion and fry gently for 8 minutes. Add the garlic and chilli and fry for a further 2 minutes.

- Stir in the chopped tomatoes, white wine, vegetable stock, bay leaf and thyme. Bring to the boil, then reduce the heat to medium–low and simmer, uncovered, for 20 minutes.

- Add the butternut squash and cook for a further 20 minutes. Stir in the butter (lima) beans.
- Preheat the oven 180°C/160°C fan/350°F/Gas mark 4. Mix the breadcrumbs, Parmesan, chopped nuts, parsley and the remaining tablespoon of oil together.
- Transfer the vegetable sauce to a suitable casserole dish and sprinkle on the crumble topping. Season liberally with salt and pepper. Bake in the oven for 30 minutes or until the crumble is golden and crisp.

Bonuses

As a special thank you for purchasing The New 5:2 Diet Cookbook, I've got some amazing bonuses to get you started.

Bonus 1: Easy Calorie Counter Cheat Sheet

So that you know whether you can have 'those little extras'

Bonus 2: Diet Day Diary

Keep track of your calories throughout the day.

Bonus 3: Bonus Recipes - Feta and Avocado Salad + Mushroom Stuffed Peppers

All these bonuses are ready and waiting for you here:

http://www.52recipes.co.uk/52bonus/

Index

D

E

F

J

L

P

Q

R

S

Salmon
  Baked Salmon With Asparagus 114
  Steamed Salmon With Spicy Rice 139
  Wasabi Salmon 116

Sausages
  Rainy Day Stew 153
  Sausage Cassoulet 165

Scallops
  Seared Scallops With Garlicky Potatoes 115

Smoothie
  Strawberry Smoothie 53

Soup
  Borscht (Chunky Beetroot Soup) 92
  Butternut Soup With Goat's Cheese 100
  Carrot And Coriander Soup 90
  Chorizo And Tomato Soup 101
  Creamy Mushroom And White Wine Soup 89
  Fresh Garden Soup 97
  Hearty Ham Soup 103
  Lentil, Lemon And Thyme Soup 102
  Mexican Chicken Soup 95
  Minestrone 105
  Roasted Parsnip Soup 93
  Savoy Cabbage And Bacon Soup 99
  Slow Onion Soup 94
  Spicy Sweet Potato Soup 91

Stews
  Beef Bourguignon 154
  Beef Pot Roast 157
  Lamb Tagine 147
  Light Chicken Stew 129
  Mixed Bean Chilli 173
  Quick Italian Beef Stew 143
  Rainy Day Stew 153
  Sausage Cassoulet 165
  Slow-Cooked Chilli Beef Stew 161
  Traditional Pork Goulash 151
  Vegetarian Bolognaise 175

Stir-fry
  Chinese Chicken Stir-Fry 125
  Pork Stir-Fry With Noodles 166

22217593R00116

Printed in Great Britain
by Amazon